NAVIGATING YOUR MIGRAINE JOURNEY

Finding a Pathway Back to Better Health

ROB WALLIS

Published by Rob Wallis
www.mymigrainementor.com.au
The moral right of the author has been asserted.

For quantity sales, speaking enquiries or media enquiries, please contact the publisher at the website address above.

ISBN: 978-1-7645455-0-1 (paperback)
978-1-7645455-1-8 (eBook)

Author photograph by *Darlene Andrews*
Graphics by *Lani Croaker*
Editing by *Kelsey Garlick*
Cover Design by *Miladinka Milic*
Interior Layout by *Olivier Darbonville*
Publishing Consultant *Linda Diggle*

NATIONAL LIBRARY OF AUSTRALIA
A catalogue record for this book is available from the National Library of Australia

To Janine

My partner in all things – life, love, family, work and fun.

Thanks for walking every part of this journey with me.

This book is as much yours as it is mine.

Contents

Foreword

It is a pleasure to write a foreword to *Navigating Your Migraine Journey: Finding a Pathway Back to Better Health*, Rob Wallis' insightful and practical book containing invaluable advice for people suffering migraine.

As a neurologist, I have worked with Rob for many years and am very grateful for his superb and professional help in the care of our patients suffering this challenging condition.

Rob's book is particularly authentic for two main reasons viz. (1) he has a wealth of experience in the management of individuals suffering migraine and (2) he has lived experience of this condition.

The traditional neurological approach to migraine has generally comprised serial poly-pharmacy with limited utility and not insignificant side-effects. No wonder patients (and doctors) found this a challenging and frustrating condition to manage.

The triptans heralded a major breakthrough in managing the symptoms of acute migraine with onabotulinum toxin and subsequently CGRP antagonists proving very helpful for the prevention of chronic migraine.

But as Rob Wallis so eloquently and thoughtfully explains, this complex syndrome demands and deserves a multifaceted holistic approach in order to empower our patients and achieve an optimal therapeutic outcome.

Comprehensive and successful management of the migraine syndrome behoves consideration of the biopsychosocial principles underpinning migraine and the many factors which may trigger or exacerbate migraine in each individual patient.

As Rob Wallis suggests, this holistic approach requires an experienced team with the patient at its epicentre and comprising the general practitioner as the primary carer and, when necessary, the neurologist providing additional specialist help; the physiotherapist; the clinical psychologist; and evidence-based complementary and natural therapists.

I often hear from patients how they have suffered migraines for many years, with significant disruption to their wellbeing and independence before being diagnosed and effectively managed. There is abundant evidence in the medical literature revealing the under-diagnosis of this common and disabling condition.

Navigating Your Migraine Journey: Finding a Pathway Back to Better Health should be widely distributed and read as it will help patients suffering migraine to recognise and understand the nature of their syndrome and receive the comprehensive and holistic treatment they need and deserve in a timely way.

Raymond Schwartz MBBS FRACP PhD
Clinical Assoc Prof. Sydney University

Author's Note

Whenever I work with clients, my aim is to help them understand the migraine process and how the science, as we currently understand it, applies to their unique situation. I have endeavoured to maintain a similar tone in this book; however, the information provided is necessarily generalised. While I have included examples to illustrate specific presentations, the content (including text and diagrams) is not intended to serve as a diagnostic tool for your migraine or as a substitute for professional medical advice and treatment.

The science of migraine is complex, and while my explanations are grounded in scientific understanding, they have been simplified to make the information more accessible and relatable. It is important to note that summarising the intricate science of migraine in a straightforward manner inevitably omits critical nuances required for accurate diagnosis and treatment. For this reason, you should always seek advice from a fully qualified medical professional who specialises in migraine and understands its complexities as a medical condition, along with the potential interventions available.

INTRODUCTION

Thriving, Not Just Surviving

It was Christmas Day, 2007. The nausea had set in. I could hear my extended family enjoying the festivities from afar. Without me. My head was over the porcelain bowl, vomiting for the 10th time. It was the third hour of another migraine attack.

This was when I personally hit rock bottom. I was 45 years old, supposedly in the prime of my life. And yet… Twenty-minute cycles of vomiting. Feeling better for a few minutes before the nausea set in again, slowly building to that climactic act. Until the only thing left to vomit was a rancid green-coloured liquid from my bile duct, my stomach empty but my migraine brain still triggering the nausea–vomiting response.

This was the third Christmas Day in five years that a migraine had struck. Another year where I lost the chance to build lifelong family memories with my young children. All I could do was hope for the sun to set and the nausea to end. In the depths of these migraine episodes my scrambled thinking floated in and out of reality – a feeling of 'disconnect' between my brain and my body. The more I experienced it, the more dehumanising and depressing it became.

Something needed to change!

Fast forward to the present. The year 2026. I am a physiotherapist, working in the headache space for over 17 years. I have heard my own experience echoed back to me, many times over. It is an all-too-familiar story:

migraine disrupting life, and the negative impact it has on physical and mental health. It is especially common for those in their thirties and forties[1] – the time when you should be enjoying your best health, raising a young family or building a career that you have worked so hard to establish. It leaves many questions unanswered.

How do I live life when this cloud of disability hangs over my head, threatening to derail the plans and goals I have for my future?

How can I stay present? Be involved in life as a partner, a parent, a family member, a co-worker, a boss, a friend?

What is the best way to approach and overcome this debilitating issue?

These very questions have led me on a journey down an unexpected path, both personally and professionally. Firstly, I had to understand what was causing my migraine disability, and secondly, I had to find solutions to my problem. Sometimes we embark on a journey out of a positive desire, but I was dragged into this by a health issue that seemed beyond my control. A disabling condition that, at times, stopped me from participating in life. Most disturbingly, it could strike at any time, without prejudice, which meant it prevented me from attending special celebrations and enjoying major life events. The reality was it impeded my ability to just 'do life'.

As a migraineur yourself, perhaps your episodes are still just a minor inconvenience … or have they become a defining aspect of your life? I use the title 'migraineur' with caution because I do not want to use a label which identifies someone as their disability. This is an issue we will address as we walk through this book. Being defined by your disability can be problematic, as it can impact your confidence and expectation to be a fully functioning member of society. It is especially difficult for those spiralling towards rock bottom, so I will use the word 'migraineur' cautiously and with respect.

The encouraging news I have to share is it is possible to understand your migraine disease and have a plan of attack to deal with it. Surprisingly, in travelling this journey myself, I didn't only reduce the severity and frequency of my migraine attacks, but I found a pathway back to better overall health. The goal of this book is to help you take control of your health and find your own individual pathway to improvement.

The Burden of Migraine

The music of your youth often becomes the playlist of your life. For me, the late '70s into the '80s was a formative time when rock music had some grunt but also a message. Bands like Midnight Oil and U2 were huge on the world stage, bringing a message that made me think more about life and my place in it. I love how these great bands can put a significant message into a few simple words. There's a song called "God Part ll" on my favourite U2 album *Rattle and Hum*, which talks about how the sick remain poor while the rich have the privilege of health. It's a message which is so applicable to migraine, because it's not just a commentary on financial wealth but on lived experience.

Migraine is often described in the literature as a complex neurological disorder. What does this mean? Essentially, it signifies that your normal brain processes tend to be disrupted. This disruption, at a microscopic level, leads to the disruption of life at a macroscopic or activity level. It has an impact on physical and mental health – an impact that can diminish at times, only to reappear for no apparent reason.

One consistent experience for all those suffering from migraine disease is the substantial impact on life, causing a poverty in life experiences. This mediocrity of life experience is not just yours alone; it's shared with those around you, restricting you and your circle of friends and family from enjoying life together.

Those who are affected by migraine stay 'poor' in numerous ways. It is more than just a financial burden, although this can be a significant part of the struggle. An Australian study in 2020 projected that over the next decade, the reduced productivity caused by migraine would cost the economy billions of dollars annually.[1] Many similar studies have been performed around the world, and they all concur [2] Migraine presents a huge health and economic burden especially because it affects people most during their productive work years.

For the person (and family) experiencing migraine disease, the limitation in earning capacity and increased medical costs are the tip of the iceberg. These costs may equate to thousands of dollars each year. [1,2] In attempting to hold down a high-demands job, an individual may find themselves working well below their normal threshold level of competence, simply to limit their stress load. This can restrict a person's earning capacity and produces feelings of inadequacy, leading to further frustration and, consequently, more stress.

Relationships and personal connections, especially within the family unit, share migraine's heavy burden. A study on families found that migraine commonly impacts an individual's ability to enjoy family activities.[3] Further strain can also be placed on the partner and children through increased domestic duties such as cleaning. Up to 40% of those experiencing migraine as a chronic condition believed their partner did not fully appreciate the severity and limitations the issue created.[3] These factors together can create real strain on relationships.

But it's not just in the family unit. The tentacles of migraine's influence can reach even further than one might expect. Cancelled social events and misconceptions of migraine disability also impact relationships with friends. The need for limitations on diet and avoidance of bright and/ or noisy venues make social times difficult to organise. Loud concerts, a time to celebrate the music we love, are often ruled out because of the sensory overload. This limitation to social interaction not only affects an individual's personal connections, but also their mental health and pain response, magnifying both issues.

It is a common experience of a person with migraine that others don't understand the issues they are facing – a truism, mostly because each individual's migraine experience is different. It is a problem that is difficult to pigeonhole, to put in a box. We like to do this with health problems because it gives us certainty and makes us feel safer. However, migraine is so experiential. Until you have gone through it, it is hard to understand. Even when you have experienced migraine, it can be difficult to describe because your brain is so scrambled by the process. Trying to explain something so complex from a health perspective can be extremely frustrating.

A major downside of this inability to describe the migraine experience is society's misunderstanding of migraine as a disease. Often people assume you just have a headache, so they perceive you are malingering, lazy or not putting in the effort. They believe all you need is a paracetamol and to get on with it. It may not be a spoken word, just inferred by actions or silence, yet this stigma can lead to further social isolation, amplifying the poverty experience.

It sounds apocalyptic, I know, but that's why we need to give the millions around the world who experience migraine every chance to improve.

Developing a Holistic Approach

I am passionate about stretching the medical model to include better health outcomes for all people who suffer migraine disease. It is important to understand this proposal. It is not replacing the present medical approach to migraine; it's adding to it! It is helping the person with migraine disease to enjoy as many of life's experiences and encounters as possible.

All the interventions outlined in this book are aimed at just that – improving the resilience of a person living with migraine so they can experience life as the best version of themselves. Not just surviving from day to day but thriving within their genetic framework, knowing what they can do to minimise the risk of triggering a severe migraine, whilst improving their health.

So, what does stretching the medical model look like? I'm sure many of you may have had a similar experience to the following scenario…

> *You have been to a medical practitioner for your headache issues and have been diagnosed with migraine. You may not have a clear understanding of what migraine is or why you are experiencing them, but you just want some relief. You have probably been offered an acute care medication which you take at the onset of an attack. Depending upon your frequency, a preventative medication, taken daily, may also have been suggested. Often these medications can be useful for a period of time but gradually lose their mojo, resulting in your migraine attacks ramping up again. A different medication may be prescribed, or perhaps an increase in dosage, which can be beneficial. This is the frustration of migraine treatment, as these medications can also take a few months to prove their usefulness.*

This one-pronged, drug-focused approach is the existing medical model. To make it clear, medications will always be important in the treatment of migraine. The types of medications used in migraine are becoming more targeted as the underlying mechanisms driving the disease are better understood, and many people benefit from their use. This is a personal choice for each person to make about their medical management.

What is missing is a recognition that migraine has significant health impacts on a person.[4] Hence, I would simply like to add a few more health-related pathways in support of people living with migraine disease, expanding the one-pronged approach into a multi-faceted treatment plan. The benefits will be improved health outcomes as well as an improvement in your migraine presentation.

In reality, it's more like widening the path, adding a few more lanes to broaden the impact we can have on migraine disease. It has been my experience, in the 40 years I have been a physiotherapist, that many people now prefer to take proactive approaches, such as lifestyle changes, to improve their health rather than rely solely on medication.

This book takes you through the journey I have been on over the past 17 years – a process of self-reflection and analysis, leading to a better understanding of my individual migraine presentation. In sharing my own experiences, my in-depth research and my physiotherapy work in the area of migraine disease, I hope to help you similarly understand your own migraine disease through a three-part process in this book.

Section 1 – Understanding the Science

You will start your journey by learning some of the complexities of what's going on in your brain when you experience a migraine attack. This area of understanding is crucial but often neglected by those in the health community treating people with migraine. This is because it is a complicated issue, and explanations can be convoluted and elaborate. While my explanations will be built on the science, it will not be an in-depth scientific exploration. A plain-English explanation is possible and can greatly enhance your attitude and approach to your condition.

Section 2 – Recognising the Triggers

Once your understanding of your migraine brain is enhanced, we will review all the possible environmental and lifestyle factors that can influence migraine. Discovering what is triggering your migraine attacks is often an ongoing source of frustration. Diet and gut issues, stress and poor sleep patterns are a few of the common triggers which often combine to contribute to your individual migraine presentation. But why do they have such a massive impact? We will journey through and break down all the possibilities, as well as looking at some less commonly accepted triggers. More importantly, we will explore why these potential triggers create problems for those with migraine disease.

Section 3 – Developing Your Individual Plan

Finally, we will review every possible intervention from a holistic point of view. You will know your options! We will navigate a simple five-step strategy to help determine the best approach for you. This aspect of intervention is crucial because it will focus on you as an individual, and your unique migraine presentation. This will allow for your own specific individual strategy. As a migraine practitioner it is rare for me to treat two people with exactly the same migraine presentation. When it happens, treatment strategies will still vary because we are all individuals and respond differently to interventions. This five-step process, when put into practice systematically, will help you determine the specific interventions that make a difference for you.

Your Healthier Future Awaits

Let's imagine a possible alternative for your future migraine treatment...

- A journey that will incorporate a holistic approach to migraine (and your health)
- A powerful combination of interventions that can have a substantial multiplying effect on your health and migraine outcomes
- Results achieved through a carefully planned and structured program tailored to your unique needs as an individual, not just as a condition

As you travel this road you will benefit from having a support team around you, a crew of medical and non-medical people, who understand your condition and can encourage and direct you back to a better place.

Due to the nature of migraine and its ability to strip you of your daily energy and drive to achieve higher goals, the thought of embarking on a new journey may seem too much to consider. If that is the case, consider this new pathway more as a 'focused wandering' rather than a 'hectic race' – a time to walk and contemplate how you can live your life to its full potential. Due to the natural variation in most migraine presentations, a slow journey is often the most effective way to approach your lifestyle factors anyway. You may want to fast-track the process, however, there is no pressure to rush through it.

If you are ready, let's start the journey together.

01

Chapter 1:

Your Genetics – It's Out of Your Control

Chapter 2:

The Migraine Brain – Migraine in Action

Chapter 3:

Migraine or Headache – Why the Confusion?

SECTION 1

The Science

CHAPTER 1

Your Genetics

It's Out of Your Control

Have you ever wondered what you did to deserve this life? Asked yourself that confronting but pertinent question: "Why is this happening to me?"

In my 17 years as a headache and migraine physiotherapist, it's a question I've heard regularly. Frustrated clients often sit across from me, grappling with the debilitating symptoms of migraine – head pain, nausea, vomiting, light and noise sensitivity. I see the unrecognised symptoms of migraine too – the loneliness, stress and social isolation that comes from living with an invisible, yet debilitating, ailment.

I once asked myself those same questions in the depths of my migraine episodes. I know the sound of those subtle internal voices telling you that in some way it's your fault. Those voices are often at their loudest when you're lying in a dark room, ice pack on your head, curtains pulled as tight as possible because any sliver of light splintering the darkness only adds to the pain. When this excruciating cycle is on repeat, the question returns: "What did I do to deserve this?"

Well, here's the answer to that ultimate question: you did nothing to deserve this. It's important that you don't blame yourself. The reality is you could probably blame your parents, or at least your ancestors. Put simply, if you have a parent or grandparent with migraine, you are more likely to have migraine yourself.

Many clients coming to our headache centres don't understand that migraine has genetic origins. Some, though, are already acutely aware of this. Their migraine history is obvious after seeing a parent experience the same debilitating effects.

Take, for example, a client I see every few months. Chelsea[1] is a 30-year-old woman who experiences a visual anomaly for 25 to 30 minutes preceding her severe migraine symptoms, referred to as a migraine with aura (MWA). She shares this very similar experience with her mother and grandmother – a problem which is somewhat manageable if it occurs when she is at home but less so if she's out and about and needs to get home safely.

Chelsea's experience is similar to that of many people living in families with migraine disease. Even witnessing a family member living through similar symptoms doesn't help deal with migraine's unpredictable nature. Not only is it frustrating for the person experiencing the migraine attacks, but also for their family and friends playing a support role.

And yet for members of other families I treat, the only commonality they share is the existence of migraine.

A strong link between migraine disease and family history has been widely recognised for many years. If you are a member of a family living with migraine disease, similar to Chelsea, this may appear obvious to you. However, it isn't always that clear-cut. Even in families where migraine is common, they can present very differently, and treatment approaches vary

---

1 Chelsea is a fictional portrayal of a typical client treated at our headache centres, designed to highlight a specific aspect of migraine presentation or treatment.

widely in their success amongst individuals. Nonetheless, many subsequent studies in genetics have proved the relationship to be true. Genetics can help us to understand all these variations in migraine presentation.

The Human Genome Project

In 2003, the Human Genome Project completed 13 years of extensive research into the mapping of the estimated 25,000 genes that form our human DNA, the building blocks of our bodies.[1] This information was then made available to researchers around the globe to aid in the research of all aspects of our health. Our understanding of migraine has greatly benefited from this research.

I first remember reading about migraine genetics in the *Sydney Morning Herald*, one day in a café behind our treatment facility in the Sydney CBD. It was 2016. The Centre for Genomics and Personalised Health, at the Queensland University of Technology (QUT), had been undergoing extensive research and investigation into the area and reported finding 36 genetic factors associated with migraine. These could be added to the previously reported eight, giving a total of 44 migraine genetic factors.

This was a pivotal 'aha' moment when I understood that unravelling the genetic underpinnings of migraine could significantly enhance treatment strategies for this challenging condition. I owe a special thanks to Dr Rob Smith from the QUT, who helped clarify some of the more intricate aspects of migraine genetics.

One key insight Dr Smith shared was the concept of genetic factors. A genetic factor refers to a variation in your DNA that increases your likelihood of experiencing a specific health condition. It's crucial to understand that these variations are not abnormalities. They are simply normal genetic differences that predispose some individuals to certain conditions, such as migraine. This is no different from people whose genetic profiles make them more susceptible to heart disease or arthritis. These variations don't make you 'abnormal', they simply make your genetics unique compared to those who don't experience migraine. The Human Genome Project has been instrumental in shedding light on these genetic variations and their role in many diseases.

Understanding the genetic basis of migraine disease is not just a scientific breakthrough, it's a practical tool for those who suffer from this condition. Knowing why you experience migraine and how your genetics have shaped your migraine brain can empower you to manage the condition more effectively. By embracing this knowledge, you can take a proactive approach to treatment and improve your quality of life.

Our Problematic Migraine History

Migraine seems to be as old as time. Ancient Egyptian writings describe migraine-like symptoms as far back as 3000 BC. Around 400 BC, Hippocrates, often referred to as the 'father of modern medicine', was the first to document migraine symptoms in a more scientific manner. He described visual disturbances and severe head pain as a cluster of symptoms, laying the groundwork for our understanding of the condition.[2]

Even in more recent history, such as the 1950s and 1960s, medical understanding of migraine was still vague. At the time, migraine attacks were often attributed to psychological causes, with the pain being classified as a psychosomatic disorder – essentially, a psychological issue manifesting as physical pain. Some of the psychological traits assigned to those living with migraine, explained in the medical literature, were extreme and unfounded, such as anal fixation or sadistic sexual tendencies.[3]

Can you imagine suffering from myriad migraine symptoms on a regular basis, and then being told that the pain was all in your head or a result of some twisted psychological condition? It's no wonder no one remembers your great-great-grandmother complaining about migraine. Perhaps this is why tracking down specifics in your family's medical history can be a challenging task, even if you have a detailed understanding of your family tree. Unfortunately, the stigma surrounding migraine persists even today.[4]

For individuals like Chelsea, who can clearly trace migraine symptoms across multiple generations, the hereditary link is obvious. However, for others, the connection may not be as apparent. While certain conditions, such as breast cancer or heart disease, are often well-remembered due to the significant medical interventions they require or the sad loss of loved ones, migraine presents a more complex picture. With its highly varied symptoms and widespread misunderstanding, even among medical professionals, the waters are muddier.

Unlike other conditions, migraine doesn't always present in the same way from one person to the next. Some individuals may experience symptoms that are entirely different from those of their parents or grandparents, making it less obvious that the migraine is hereditary.

The *International Classification of Headache Disorders, 3rd edition (ICHD-3)* highlights these differences.[5] It is the benchmark for classifying headache types, identifying six main categories of migraine, shown in Table 1, which are further divided into 23 sub-types. Despite this extensive classification system, it remains rare for two individuals to experience migraine in exactly the same way. One person may have a different set of symptoms with each episode, while another may experience a consistent pattern with every attack.

Table 1. Migraine Categories[5] in ICHD-3

Category	Description
Migraine without aura	The migraine starts without any major warning sign
Migraine with aura	The migraine starts with some sensation, usually visual anomaly some 30 minutes before the headache
Chronic migraine	Occurs with 15 headache days/month of which 8 have a migraine presentation
Complications of migraine	A more persistent problem related to a number of potential accompanying symptoms
Probable migraine	Doesn't quite fit the migraine criteria but looks very similar to a migraine
Episodic syndromes that may be associated with migraine	Persistent problems with gut disruption, vomiting, dizziness or neck issues without the headache pain

Not only can migraine present very differently amongst family members, there's also the added challenge of the 'knowledge factor'. Put simply, if you think a past generation in your family tree hasn't had migraine, you probably just don't know enough about your ancestors' experience.

Migraine has long been misunderstood. A key characteristic of the disorder is its ability to mimic other illnesses, making it notoriously difficult to diagnose. If migraine is difficult to diagnose today, imagine how difficult it would have been in past generations, and indeed in past centuries.

Additionally, many of our parents' or grandparents' generation lived through serious economic times – consider: world wars and the Great Depression. As a result of the times they were living in and the challenges they faced on a daily basis, they developed a 'suck-it-up' mentality, simply living with the consequences of migraine – resting in solitude when they could, getting on with life when they were able.

For the sake of all those experiencing migraine disease, a greater understanding of the causes and drivers was desperately needed. Improved brain scanning and research protocols that have been developed over the past 20 to 30 years have helped our understanding of the brain and its neurological processes. When combined with insights from the Human Genome Project, these developments have shed light on the genetic factors that contribute to the wide variations in migraine presentations. This progress offers hope for better diagnosis, treatment and understanding of migraine as a disease.

Our Predisposition to Migraine

Many of us will understand the basics of genetics. Our distinctive features are passed on to us by our parents and their family lines through our DNA. Consequently, our physical and psychological characteristics are often similar to those of our ancestors, some more evident than others. The combination of genetics from two different family lines means that while we share certain traits with our parents, we are not exactly the same. For better or for worse we do share some but not all the same features.

This includes many aspects of our health. The problem is that when genes are passed from parent to child, certain health conditions can also be inherited. The genetic DNA a child receives from both parents determines whether they are more or less prone to specific health issues, depending on the genetic combinations. This is referred to as a predisposition.

For example, if one parent has a genetic predisposition to migraine, it can be passed on to their child. This principle applies to many diseases and health conditions and has been extensively studied, often using groups of identical and non-identical twins. Research shows that if you have a parent or grandparent who experiences migraine, you are four times more likely than the general population to develop migraine disease as well.[6-9]

However, even if a parent experiences migraine, it does not guarantee that their child will develop migraine disease. For instance, I have a non-identical twin brother, John, who only experiences occasional headaches and has never had a migraine episode. When it comes to my two sisters, Lyn has never had headaches, while Liz has experienced headaches over the years. For a brief period in her life, Liz reported about six migraine episodes, and on a few occasions she required an injection to manage severe nausea. Compared to my three siblings, it seems I inherited the strongest genetic predisposition to migraine.

If you recall your high school science classes, you might remember that the genetic DNA in each cell of your body is responsible for producing proteins that regulate every aspect of your body's functioning. The goal of genetic research is to identify these key proteins and understand their impact on the body. Medical researchers have discovered that studying twins provides a valuable opportunity to better understand the role of genetics in a variety of health problems.

Twin studies gained significant attention in the 1990s – my brother and I participated in some of these studies related to mental health. The studies compared identical and non-identical twins who grew up in the same household as well as those who were separated during their early years. By analysing the health issues experienced by these twins, researchers were able to distinguish between the effects of nature (shared genetics) and nurture (lifestyle factors) on specific health conditions.

Studies on migraine confirmed the role of hereditary factors. Early research revealed that migraine was passed on to children 35–70% of the time,[7] a measure known as heritability. More recent studies indicate that heritability varies depending on the type of migraine a person experiences.

The Role of Genetics in Migraine Variations

Genetic studies aim to deepen our understanding of why an individual's migraine manifests in a specific way. The genetics of migraine can be broadly divided into two main categories: monogenic (migraine caused by a single genetic factor) or polygenic (migraine influenced by multiple genetic factors).

These categories reflect the number of individual genes involved and how they contribute to a person's unique migraine presentation. Additionally, migraine within these categories can be further classified based on the frequency of their attacks: episodic (less frequent) or chronic (occurring regularly).

Monogenic Migraine

Monogenic migraine is among the rarer forms, such as migraine with aura (MWA) or hemiplegic migraine, where a person can appear to be experiencing a stroke. These migraine types are caused by a single genetic factor that significantly influences their presentation, often making them highly disabling.

Since only one genetic factor is involved, monogenic migraine presentations have a higher likelihood of being passed from parent to child. This means the child is more likely to experience migraine in a similar way to the parent. Hemiplegic migraine is a prime example of this type. As it causes a temporary loss of function on one side of the body, mimicking the symptoms of a stroke, experiencing this for the first time can be alarming.

However, due to its strong inheritability (up to 70–90% of the time), many individuals are aware of the condition because a parent or grandparent has also experienced it.

This was not the case, though, for one of my patients, a young woman in her early twenties. She was severely affected by hemiplegic migraine, to the point where her parents felt as though they had lost their daughter. As the first in her family to experience this type of migraine, the impact on her life (and her family's) was profound and challenging for everyone to understand and adapt to. It's understandable that in cases like this, a person can quickly become defined by their disability.

Polygenic Migraine

Polygenic migraine is influenced by multiple genetic factors – potentially up to 44 – and is present in over 60% of those who experience migraine. As each genetic factor seems to have a small effect on migraine presentation, it goes part of the way to explain why every person's migraine presentation is unique. Theoretically, the variety of combinations makes it less likely for two people (even in a parent–child situation) to have the same presentation.

The complexity of polygenic migraine lies in these 44 potential contributing factors. These genetic variations lead to the production of problematic proteins that can disrupt multiple processes or chemical reactions in the body, increasing susceptibility to migraine. This intricate interplay of factors makes polygenic migraine more challenging to understand and manage.

Dr Smith notes that although there are presently 44 genetic factors accepted as migraine specific, there are possibly a lot more, potentially into the hundreds, to be unveiled.[8] These are more difficult to determine because some are only relevant if another genetic factor is present. Some genetic variations do not cause migraine themselves but can potentially increase your sensitivity to triggers.

Given the multitude of known and unknown genetic factors influencing migraine presentation, researchers like Dr Smith and the team at QUT face a significant challenge in mapping the genetic pathways behind migraine disease. However, each new discovery brings us closer to understanding the underlying mechanisms, offering hope for more effective and targeted treatment options in the future.

Episodic and Chronic Migraine

A key characteristic of both monogenic and polygenic migraine disease is the frequency of episodes over time. Migraine typically starts as an episodic condition, where a person experiences individual episodes that may last several hours or even days, followed by periods of normalcy. However, some individuals endure migraine so frequently that life becomes a continuous battle. These individuals are often referred to as 'migraine warriors' due to their relentless struggle to navigate daily life. This is known as chronic migraine, a condition defined by experiencing at least 15 headache days per month, with at least eight of those days involving migraine-like symptoms.[5]

Interestingly, the frequency of migraine is not directly tied to the number of genetic factors a person has. In other words, having 20 genetic factors does not automatically increase the risk of developing chronic migraine compared to having 10. Rather, it's the type of genetic factors in a person's DNA that matters. Dr Smith explains, "It seems likely that whether someone develops chronic migraine is determined by the specific combination of genetic variants they carry."

This genetic complexity sheds light on why migraine affects individuals so differently. As we will discuss, lifestyle and environmental factors interact with our genetic makeup and often exacerbate migraine symptoms.[10]

For instance, someone with a less potent combination of genetic factors may only experience a few migraine attacks each year, resulting in a relatively low impact on their life. In contrast, an individual with a more potent genetic combination – one that is more sensitive to external lifestyle and environmental triggers – may suffer more frequent and intense migraine attacks. These individuals are often severely impacted by their condition and face higher levels of disability related to their migraine disease. These are the true 'migraine warriors' – individuals who, through no fault of their own, are locked in a constant battle with their migraine-prone brains. Their situation is far from enviable, as they navigate a daily struggle that many cannot fully comprehend.

Genetics and Your Migraine Brain

One of the key benefits of genetic studies is their ability to shed light on the causes of migraine pain and its associated symptoms. For years, there has been debate over whether migraine stems from issues with nerves or blood vessels, both of which work together to produce the brain's remarkable abilities. What we do know is that poor functioning of nerve fibres plays a significant role in the migraine experience.

The human brain contains an estimated 80 billion individual nerve fibres. To put that into perspective, even if you counted as quickly as possible without breaks, it would take over 30 years to reach just one billion, making it impossible to count to 80 billion in a lifetime! This highlights why significant issues arise when the brain's nerve fibre function is impaired.

Although the brain accounts for only 2% of our body weight, it uses 15–20% of our blood flow and 25% of the body's total energy. There is a very close relationship between nerves and blood vessels in the brain and there has been much debate for many years over which structure causes the migraine. When it comes to the pain and symptoms of migraine, it appears that both nerves and blood vessels play a role.

It is widely accepted, though, that migraine is primarily a neurological condition caused by heightened nerve sensitivity. However, this doesn't mean that blood vessels are not involved in the pain. Changes in blood flow through these vessels is thought to be one of the pain-causing mechanisms in migraine. It's actually not surprising, as both systems are interconnected.

At a basic level, nerves control blood vessel function, and nerves themselves are highly vascular structures. Due to their complex functions, nerves have high energy demands, requiring a steady supply of blood flow to meet those energy needs. During a migraine attack, when nerves become overly sensitive, this delicate balance between energy supply and usage is disrupted, contributing to the symptoms experienced.

For more information on this topic, read ***Exploring the Science: Migraine Brain Activity.***

EXPLORING THE SCIENCE

Migraine Brain Activity

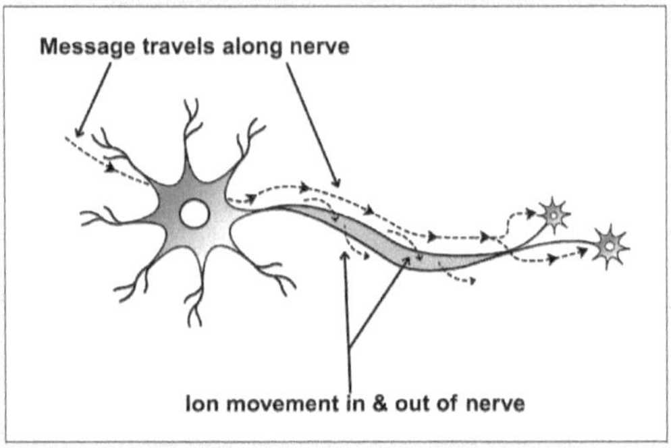

During brain activity, messages travel along individual nerve fibres via a nerve impulse caused by the movement of ions such as potassium (K), sodium (Na) and calcium (Ca). After an impulse travels along the nerve, these chemicals are then pumped back into their correct positions. This process requires a lot of energy, explaining why the brain needs high levels of blood flow to maintain its ability to process information continuously.

In a migraine-prone brain, individual nerve fibres do not function as they should. Some of the abnormal proteins we discussed earlier can cause an excessive influx of ions into the nerve fibres, disrupting the way these nerves send messages. The movement of ions within nerve and vascular tissues, along with neurotransmitters responsible for carrying messages between nerves, are also affected.

This dysfunction in ions and proteins triggers a cascade of messages being sent along the nerve fibres, leading to excessive 'excitation' in the nerves. This phenomenon, known as 'sensitisation', occurs when nerves send too many messages too quickly, overwhelming the system.

Now, imagine this process multiplied by 80 billion nerve fibres. It's easy to see how the brain, flooded with an overload of messages, becomes fatigued – a sensation all too familiar to those who experience migraine.

Considering the numerous genetic factors that influence both the neurological and vascular systems of the brain, it becomes clear why migraine is such a complex condition. This complexity also explains why treating migraine on an individual basis can be so challenging. With so many unknown variables at play, finding a single solution to completely eliminate your migraine attacks is highly unlikely.

The most effective approach is to develop a comprehensive plan that addresses the multiple factors involved in your migraine. This plan should go beyond simply relying on medications. Instead, it should include a variety of interventions that target both the neurological and vascular components contributing to your condition.

Another critical factor in creating an effective migraine treatment plan is recognising the presence of other health issues that may influence your migraine disease. By taking a holistic approach that considers all contributing factors, we can work towards reducing the impact of migraine days and improving your overall quality of life.

Comorbidities Associated with Migraine

It is worth noting that many people who experience migraine will also face other health issues more commonly than the general population. When this occurs, it is called comorbidity, and it can happen for a number of reasons related to your genetics. Having a clear understanding of this will be important when it comes to formulating your plan to 'push back' on migraine impacting your life.

Genetic studies frequently reveal shared genetic factors that increase the likelihood of a person experiencing both migraine and other conditions. There is often a positive correlation between migraine and a range of physical and psychological disorders,[2,11,12] as shown in Table 2.

Table 2. Comorbidities Associated with Migraine

DISORDER	COMORBIDITY
Psychological	Anxiety, depression, eating disorders, PTSD, ADHD
Sleep	Insomnia, frequent waking, trouble falling asleep
Autoimmune	Psoriasis, rheumatoid arthritis
Cardiovascular	Angina, heart attacks, stroke
Neurological disease	Epilepsy, multiple sclerosis, fibromyalgia, restless leg syndrome
Allergies	Sinus, hay fever
Hormonal	Hypothyroidism
Gastrointestinal	Irritable bowel syndrome, celiac disease, ulcers
Metabolic	Obesity, hypertension, high cholesterol
Reproductive	Endometriosis
Connective tissue	Ehlers-Danlos syndrome
Childhood Comorbidities	Obesity, ADHD, epilepsy, sleep disorders, allergy-related symptoms such as sinusitis

Recognising these comorbidities allows you to incorporate them into your intervention plan, as outlined in Section 3 of this book. Being aware that migraine may predispose you to other health conditions empowers you to take proactive steps to maintain good health and minimise the impact of these conditions before they lead to serious complications.

For instance, if you have a family history of type 2 diabetes or vascular disease in addition to migraine, it becomes essential to adopt a healthy diet and lifestyle. These measures can help reduce the risk of these conditions causing significant health issues in the future.

My Comorbidities

In my own family, high cholesterol and vascular disease have always been a significant concern. My maternal grandmother passed away from a stroke at the age of 67, and my paternal grandmother suffered a heart attack at 85. My father experienced two near-fatal heart attacks, one at 58 and another at 86. As a person with migraine disease, knowing that I am predisposed to high cholesterol and vascular disease as comorbidities made it a critical issue for me to address.

The encouraging news is that making healthy lifestyle changes not only reduces the risk of developing these health conditions but can also improve your migraine symptoms. Understanding your potential health risks is a vital first step. Start by journalling any health issues that run in your family. The list of possible comorbidities is extensive, so you may need to research and consult with family members to identify all relevant conditions.

Conclusion

The main takeaway message from this chapter is that migraine has a genetic foundation, something beyond your control. You were born with a brain that is naturally predisposed for migraine. So, in those dark moments when the medications are working hard to bring some relief and the ice pack feels like your closest ally, don't listen to the inner voices trying to blame you for your situation.

Still, while genetics play a role, they are only part of the story. It's difficult to pinpoint exactly how much your genetic makeup influences your health, but it's crucial to understand that it's not the sole determinant. The daily choices you make are the most significant factors in shaping your health.

Research indicates that adopting a proactive approach – incorporating lifestyle adjustments and evidence-based strategies – can significantly enhance health outcomes. Although these changes require time and patience, many individuals report feeling more empowered and in control of their health and overall wellbeing through this method.

Ultimately, the key to taking back control lies in understanding your migraine brain.

CHAPTER 2

The Migraine Brain

Migraine in Action

Neuroscience, the study of how the brain functions, is one of the most complex areas of science to comprehend. It stands alongside rocket science and the study of the universe in terms of difficulty. One of the challenges lies in the sheer magnitude of the numbers involved.

Our corner of the universe, the Milky Way, is estimated to contain over 100 billion stars spread across trillions of kilometres. Comparatively, the human brain contains approximately 80 billion individual nerve fibres, along with another trillion supporting cells, all compacted into an area roughly the size of a 1.5-litre drink bottle. The brain is thought to have a storage capacity of 2.5 million gigabytes, which, according to Google, equates to about 300 years' worth of TV programs. These figures are comparable to the vastness of the universe, yet the brain operates on the opposite end of the size spectrum. Despite its small dimensions, its capacity to process information is extraordinary. It's no surprise that so many scientists are dedicated to uncovering its mysteries.

Gaining even a basic understanding of how your brain functions and what is happening during a migraine episode can be a crucial step in regaining some control over your life. This knowledge becomes a powerful tool in your journey to reduce the impact of migraine, not only on your worst days but every day. Even on the days you are feeling great, migraine's pervasive tentacles are hovering around in your head, making it difficult to feel relaxed and free.

As you explore new pathways to improved health, accompanied by your support team, the frustrations will settle. Implementing strategies that provide a greater sense of control and direction in your journey towards better physical and mental health empowers you to reclaim your life. Understanding the origins of your symptoms is a key element in this process.

The Brainstem Region

Research into genetics suggests that migraine is linked to an increased sensitivity in the central nervous system (CNS). The CNS comprises the brain and spinal cord, but in the case of migraine, the issue is primarily centred in the brain, particularly in its lower regions. To simplify the discussion, we can divide the brain into three sections (see Figure 1). When we think of the brain, we often picture the topmost area, the cortex. This is the 'conscious' part of the brain, responsible for processing information received from the body and planning responses to that information.

There are, however, more primitive parts of the brain that function at a nonconscious level. These include the limbic system and the brainstem. The limbic system is a collection of key brain areas, including the hypothalamus and amygdala, which have a strong relationship with migraine. This region is responsible for emotional regulation, responses to environmental stress and the processing of smell.

Figure 1. Diagram of the Brain

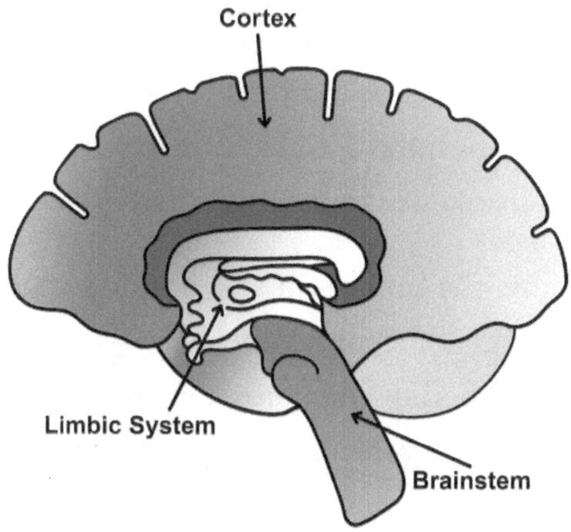

The cortex, the conscious part of the brain responsible for processing and action; the limbic system, the nonconscious part of the brain responsible for receiving sensation, processing and action.

The brainstem, on the other hand, acts as the primary gateway to the brain. Sensory information from the body passes through the brainstem before being relayed to other areas of the brain for further processing. Messages also travel from the brain, through the brainstem out to the body so we can interact with the environment around us. The brainstem region also controls many of the body's essential 'automatic' functions, such as heart rate and breathing, which occur without conscious effort. Together with the limbic system, these nonconscious areas of the brain manage functions critical to our survival. This brain region's importance is made obvious when the area is impaired with lack of blood flow.

Recently, a good mate of mine experienced a brainstem stroke. It is one of the most devastating forms of stroke, with a death rate upwards of 80%. Due to a number of factors, including early detection at the starting point of the stroke by his wife, a rapid ambulance response and timely administration of clot-dissolving medication, he survived and has made a full recovery. It wasn't lost on him how incredibly lucky he was to survive. When he was discharged from hospital several days later, his specialist walked him out of the hospital door because it was such a rare occurrence to have someone fully recover from a brainstem stroke.

It shows exactly how the brainstem and limbic system are involved in important life-sustaining functions. When you understand how the brainstem controls essential bodily functions, such as heart rate and breathing, whether you are awake or asleep, you can understand why it has been called 'the stem of life'.[1]

When a migraine attack hits, it increases the sensitivity of the nerves of the brain and has a major impact on the brainstem region. Due to this I often refer to the brainstem as the 'centre of the migraine universe'. It's no wonder migraine creates so many issues that affect our quality of life.

An Over-Reactive Computer Hub

The brainstem can be likened to a highly efficient computer hub that keeps your body running smoothly without conscious effort. Just as a smart home system turns the lights on and off, sets the air-conditioning to the perfect temperature and reminds you when you have an appointment coming up, the brainstem is similar. It receives information from the body and other parts of the brain, reacting automatically to maintain optimal function. For example, it regulates your heart and breathing rates to ensure your body gets the oxygen it needs, especially during exercise. This vital region, along with the limbic system, is essential for survival.

For individuals without migraine, this 'control hub' operates seamlessly, ensuring that nerve pathways deliver messages efficiently. However, for those with migraine disease, the brainstem becomes overly reactive during an attack. This heightened reactivity, known as central sensitisation, disrupts the nerve pathways, causing the brainstem to malfunction. It's as if the computer hub in your house starts flickering the lights, overheating the room and forgetting to remind you of your next neurologist appointment. This dysfunction significantly impacts the quality of life for those living with migraine disease. This inherent characteristic of reactivity makes the migraine brain respond to normal sensations in an unusual way, hence creating all the extraordinary symptoms.

Understanding the brainstem's role and the concept of central sensitisation provides valuable insight into why migraine is so debilitating and why effective management is crucial for improving the lives of those affected.

The Reason for the Symptoms

Migraine causes a range of disabling symptoms that may appear unrelated, such as noise sensitivity, nausea, neck pain, fatigue or dizziness. The connection lies within the brainstem and the 12 cranial nerves, shown in Figure 3, which transmit signals between the brain, head and gut.

Figure 2. The 12 Cranial Nerves' Entry Points

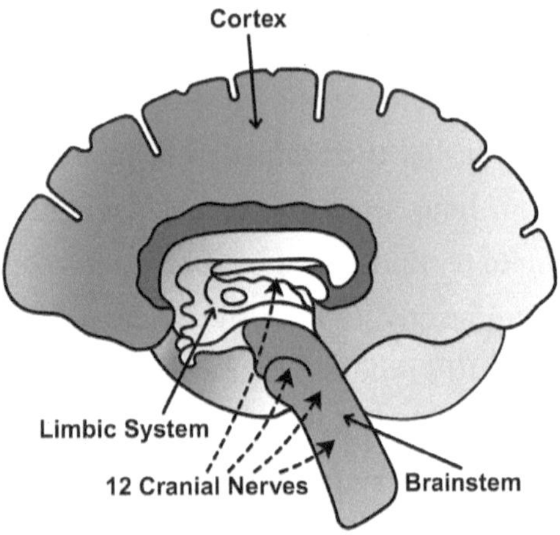

The cranial nerves enter into the brain via the brainstem, except for #1 which enters through the limbic region.

These 12 nerves travel directly through the brainstem and limbic regions. They are responsible for controlling many important functions necessary for our survival including sight, smell, digestion and cardiovascular function, as shown in Table 3.

Table 3. The 12 Cranial Nerves and Their Functions

Cranial Nerve	Name	Function
#1	Olfactory	Sinus innervation and sense of smell
#2	Optic	Eye nerve for vision
#3	Oculomotor	Muscles for eye movement and focus
#4	Trochlea	Muscle for eye movement
#5	Trigeminal	Sensation to top of head and face, jaw muscles for chewing
#6	Abducens	Muscle for eye movement
#7	Facial	Muscles of face, mouth and head, taste to front 2/3 of tongue and glands for mouth/saliva and tears
#8	Vestibulocochlear	Ear nerve for hearing and balance
#9	Glossopharyngeal	Taste to back 1/3 of tongue, sensation in throat and middle ear, swallowing and gag reflex
#10	Vagus	Motor function of the heart, lungs, gut, lower throat. Sensation for the external ear, heart, lungs, gut and throat
#11	Accessory	Sternocleidomastoid and upper trapezius (neck) muscles
#12	Hypoglossal	Tongue muscles

However, when the brainstem becomes overactive, it disrupts these functions, consequently triggering a wide array of migraine symptoms. As this lower part of the brain becomes increasingly sensitive, the symptoms can vary significantly within or between episodes.

When you examine the functions associated with each cranial nerve in Table 4, you may recognise many symptoms familiar to your migraine episodes. During a migraine, the sensitised brainstem disrupts and amplifies the messages passing through it. This heightened reactivity leads to the diverse and often debilitating symptoms you experience.

Table 4. Potential Symptoms Driven by the Cranial Nerves

Cranial Nerve	Potential Symptom
#1	Sinus irritation or a blocked feeling, smell sensitivity
#2	Disruption to normal field of vision, light sensitivity
#3 #4 #6	Strained feeling in eyes or blurry vision
#5	Pain in the teeth, jaw, face or top of head, teeth grinding (often at night)
#7	Muscle tension or paralysis in face
#8	Dizziness, balance problems, noise sensitivity
#9 #12	Difficulty swallowing
#10	Nausea and vomiting, racing heart rate, breathing issues
#11	Neck muscle pain and tightness in neck and shoulders

Migraine the Mimic

One of the more perplexing aspects of a reactive, hypersensitive brainstem and the connecting cranial nerves is their ability to produce symptoms that closely resemble those of other common health conditions. Migraine can mimic a variety of issues, including gut, sinus, visual or balance problems, as well as other headache disorders. This often leads health professionals astray when attempting to establish a diagnosis. The mimicry occurs because the heightened reactivity of the nerves generates symptoms of conditions that are not actually present. These pseudo-symptoms can be particularly frustrating, as they often prompt doctors to order tests or refer patients to specialists, only for the results to come back inconclusive. Many patients are left hearing statements like, "We can't find any problems with your vision, hearing, gut, etc."

Take, for example, one of my clients, Gary[2]. He experienced intermittent blurry vision, prompting his doctor to refer him to an optometrist, who found no issues with his eyes. This was followed by scans of his brain to rule out a tumour. With no clear explanation for his symptoms, Gary was left puzzled until he noticed a pattern. His blurry vision coincided with other subtle migraine symptoms, such as mild light and noise sensitivity and a vague sense of disorientation. In reality, his blurry vision was likely caused by migraine disrupting the messages travelling between his eyes and brain via the brainstem.

There is a particular type of migraine that is characterised by recurring episodes of nausea and vomiting, without the presence of a headache or other typical migraine symptoms. Called cyclic vomiting syndrome (CVS), it can be deeply confusing for both the individual and their medical practitioners until a correct diagnosis is made. A variety of tests for the gut will show no issues and can take up significant time. Once the initial diagnosis and classification of CVS is made, effective management can be established.

It is not uncommon for people who visit our headache centres to report having already consulted multiple specialists. Many have seen an optometrist, only to be told they have perfect 20/20 vision. Others have undergone extensive testing with a gastroenterologist for nausea or frequent vomiting, only to receive the 'all clear'. Some have consulted an ENT (ear, nose and

---

2 Gary is a fictional representation of a typical client we treat in our headache centres, used to amplify a specific aspect of migraine presentation or treatment.

throat) or vestibular specialist for dizziness, only to be informed that everything is functioning normally. This often results in the classic "Nothing to see here, move along now" response. When this happens repeatedly, it can lead to significant psychological frustration, which may exacerbate the symptoms.

As frustrating as this process is for the person with migraine, it is also a difficult position for doctors. They feel a responsibility to investigate all possible causes of your symptoms, as missing a critical diagnosis could have serious consequences. At the same time, they are often aware of your growing frustration when test results repeatedly come back with the 'all clear' tag.

A final, and somewhat contrary, point is that chronic migraine over an extended period can, in some cases, lead to the development of an actual disease process in the body. For instance, frequent migraine episodes that cause persistent nausea and vomiting may eventually result in significant gut dysfunction. The body struggles to cope with such ongoing disruption, which can lead to the need for more specialised treatment to address the resulting issues. Although this is more the exception than the rule, it emphasises the importance of being proactive with your approach to the disease.

The Migraine Brain

Migraine is influenced by a genetic predisposition, causing parts of the brain, including the brainstem, to become hypersensitive to normal sensory input due to sensitisation. In cases of episodic migraine, which is more common, the brain typically returns to normal functioning between attacks. During these periods, the nerve pathways calm down, allowing you to feel like your true self. However, during a migraine attack, the brain enters an altered, sensitised state, making you feel far from normal.

For individuals experiencing chronic migraine – defined as migraine attacks occurring at least eight days each month – the brain often remains in a prolonged sensitised state. In some cases, this leads to a persistent cycle of heightened sensitivity.

Regardless of whether you experience episodic or chronic migraine, it is crucial to acknowledge that the psychological impact of the condition can be ever-present, affecting emotional wellbeing and quality of life.

Brain Connections and Sensitisation

The brain's ability to share information across different regions is due to a remarkable feature known as functional connectivity. This intricate process allows the brainstem to communicate seamlessly with other areas, such as the limbic system and cortex (see Figure 3), enabling the brain to process information at higher, more complex levels. Functional connectivity ensures the brain operates efficiently, maintaining coordination and balance across its networks.

However, when this connectivity is disrupted, as often happens during a migraine, the ripple effects can impair the brain's ability to function normally. It is akin to the brain running an error message, which affects your ability to function as you usually would, affecting everything from pain regulation to emotional responses. Research indicates that there is no single, consistent pattern of overactivity during every migraine, which explains why each individual migraine can present with different characteristics[2] – and why they're so debilitating.

Similarly, cortical spreading depression (CSD) plays a pivotal role in the profound effects of migraine on brain function. CSD is a wave of intense nerve cell activity followed by a period of inactivity, caused by an imbalance in sodium, potassium and calcium ions within the brain's messaging system. Essentially, the nerve cells become unable to send messages as they normally would. It is comparable to running a 400-metre race and collapsing at the finish line, requiring a prolonged recovery period. This process disrupts normal nerve communication, leaving the brain in a state of temporary dysfunction. CSD is often linked to the visual aura some people experience before migraine pain, but it can occur at various stages of a migraine episode. Its effects are not limited to one area; CSD can spread from the brainstem to higher brain regions, amplifying the impact of migraine on cognitive and physical abilities.

Figure 3. Brain Connections

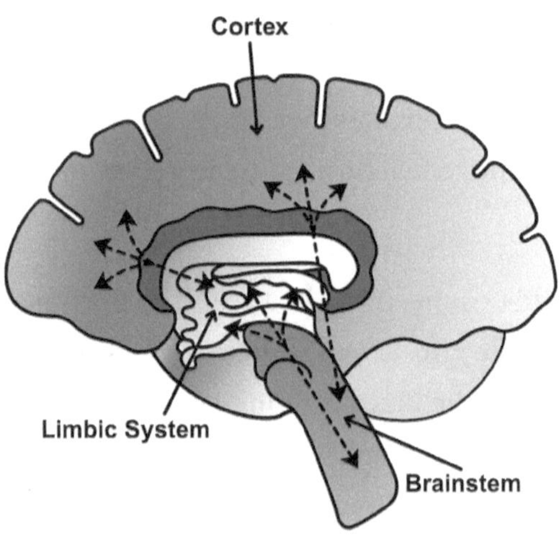

Connections between the brainstem, limbic system and cortex.

Together, functional connectivity and CSD illustrate the complex and far-reaching nature of migraine. It should now be evident why migraine can significantly limit your ability to function in daily life. The disruption of countless nerve pathways at a microscopic level significantly limits your body's ability to tolerate daily activities – the pathways you navigate in your day-to-day life.

The Migraine Threshold

What lies behind the ebb and flow of migraine? This is best explained by a concept known as the 'migraine threshold'. Over the years, as research has advanced our understanding of the migraine brain, researchers have developed the concept of the 'migraine threshold'. This threshold represents the theoretical level of sensitivity that must be reached before a migraine is triggered. It is a concept that helps explain, in part, why you are not always in a migraine state. Sensitivity levels in the brain fluctuate daily and can be influenced by a variety of environmental or lifestyle factors.

For individuals who experience episodic or occasional migraine, their brain can function 'normally' most of the time. However, when the central nervous system (CNS) reaches a certain level of sensitivity, a migraine is triggered. Studies have demonstrated significant involvement of multiple brain regions, including the brainstem, limbic system (hypothalamus, amygdala, thalamus), prefrontal cortex and visual system, as migraine develops.[2-9]

The theory of the migraine threshold can be illustrated in several ways. Common analogies include 'a bucket being filled to the point of overflowing' or 'a computer hub overloading and blowing a circuit'. Personally, I prefer to use a graph, like Figure 4 below, to explain this concept to my patients, as it provides a clear visual representation of how sensitivity levels fluctuate and how triggers can push the brain over the threshold.

Figure 4. Migraine Threshold Graph

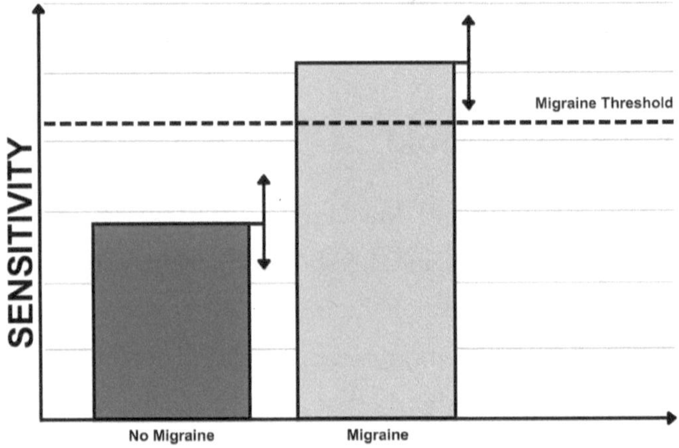

Our nerve sensitivity levels tend to vary on an ongoing basis. A migraine will occur when a person's sensitivity reaches threshold level.

Stages of a Migraine

Once you reach your migraine threshold, you enter the familiar territory of the migraine itself. While each individual migraine episode can develop different characteristics over time (as various parts of the brain are affected), the basic structure of a migraine will likely remain recognisable to you.

The migraine process is generally divided into four basic phases, each associated with specific symptoms. These phases do not always occur in a strict sequence, so it's important not to expect distinct patterns every time. However, over time, you may notice recurring patterns that help you better understand what is happening in your brain.[3]

Most educational resources about migraine define these four stages using common terminology. Familiarising yourself with these terms can provide clarity when navigating the often confusing symptoms of migraine.

Premonitory Phase

This phase can occur hours or even days before the onset of pain. Symptoms are often subtle and may be mistaken for normal variations in daily life. Commonly reported symptoms include drowsiness, yawning, irritability, fatigue, nausea, food cravings, frequent urination, poor concentration, mood changes, and neck pain. It is believed that this phase originates in the hypothalamus region of the limbic system.[3,4]

Early recognition of the premonitory phase may allow for timely intervention to prevent a migraine headache from developing. However, identifying consistent patterns may take time. Keeping a journal can help you confirm the symptoms associated with this phase. One challenge is distinguishing whether symptoms such as anxiety or neck pain are part of the premonitory phase or triggers for the migraine episode.

Aura Phase (only 30% of people)

The aura phase typically lasts around 30 minutes (ranging from 5 to 60 minutes) before the headache phase begins. In 90% of cases, it involves visual disturbances such as flashing lights, wavy lines or temporary vision loss. Other aura symptoms may include numbness or tingling in the body or limbs, speech difficulties or uncoordinated movements. Cortical spreading depression (CSD) is thought to play a significant role in driving the aura phase.

Headache Phase

This is the phase most people dread. The headache can be one-sided (60% of cases) or affect both sides of the head (40%). It is often described as throbbing or pulsating, although this occurs in only 50% of cases. The headache typically takes about an hour to reach full intensity and is often described as moderate to severe. Neck pain is a common symptom during this phase. Other associated symptoms include sensitivity to light and noise, dizziness, nausea and vomiting, which frequently accompany the headache phase.

Postdrome Phase

This 'after-the-headache' phase occurs in 80% of people and begins as the headache subsides. Often referred to as the 'migraine hangover', this is essentially a recovery period during which the brain recharges. Symptoms during this phase may include fatigue, sleepiness, nausea, irritability and difficulty concentrating. The postdrome phase can last up to 24 hours as the nerves take time to restore normal energy levels within the cells to function properly again.

The Interictal Period – Between Migraine Episodes

The interictal period is the time between migraine episodes when the individual feels essentially normal. However, even during this phase, the person may remain more sensitive than usual to sensory stimuli.

It's important to note that these phases are not consistent for every migraine episode. They often overlap and can vary significantly between attacks. These classifications are intended to provide a practical framework for understanding migraine episodes and should not be used for making a specific diagnosis.[3,4]

Migraine Pain

What remains consistent for all migraine attacks is the disabling nature of the pain. When it comes to the headache phase, migraine pain feels distinct from other types of pain and often seems more challenging to endure. Does this resonate with you? It certainly did with me.

My Pain Experience

I have always been an active person, participating in various sports and generally managing injuries and pain quite well. A good example of this was during my childhood when I required extensive dental work. My father was a dentist, and I wasn't exactly the best advertisement for his skills, as a childhood illness left me with terrible teeth. As a result, I frequently needed fillings and other dental procedures. While I coped well with the dental work itself, I despised the local anaesthetic, which left me drooling and uncomfortable for hours.

On one occasion, my father needed to perform some minor drilling to clean up a small area of decay. He asked if I wanted to try the procedure without local anaesthetic, and I agreed. Surprisingly, I managed reasonably well. I stayed calm and found the pain tolerable. Of course, I wouldn't attempt the same for something like a root canal, but this experience highlighted my ability to handle a certain level of pain and discomfort.

However, when I began experiencing migraine pain, it was an entirely different story. I vividly recall one Christmas Day, lying on the bathroom floor with my forehead pressed against the cool tiles, desperately seeking relief. I remember repeatedly asking myself, "What is going on?" – a strange question in hindsight, as I knew exactly what was happening. The real issue seemed to be my brain's inability to process the situation rationally.

This is the challenging nature of migraine pain. It seems to stem from the disruption caused to the brain's higher centres, particularly the prefrontal cortex (PFC). The PFC, located in the front part of the brain's cortex, plays a crucial role in the cognitive appraisal of pain. It is part of the brain's conscious planning and control centre, enabling us to respond to life's challenges in a measured way – it enables us to stay connected to the reality of our situation. Interestingly, the PFC is one of the last areas of the brain to fully develop, especially in males.

When CSD affects the PFC and severely inhibits its function, it can impair your ability to rationally process migraine pain. This disruption does not occur in the same way during a typical acute injury. If migraine becomes more chronic, the functional connectivity of the brain's pain-processing networks is further compromised, leading to increased sensitisation. As a result, your response to pain may become more confused and irrational. For individuals living with chronic migraine, life can become incredibly challenging. Their brains are perpetually exhausted, leaving them physically and emotionally drained.

This is where the amygdala, a small but vital part of the brain, may play a role. Named after the Greek word for 'almond' due to its shape, the amygdala is involved in memory processing, decision making and emotional responses. It has strong connections with the PFC and can influence how we emotionally respond to pain. If the amygdala is affected by migraine processes, it seems plausible that your ability to cope with pain is further diminished. Research has suggested that this may also be the case in paediatric migraine,[10] indicating that these processes can begin early in life.

From my own experience with migraine pain and my understanding of the research, I believe that when the brain's higher executive functions are compromised, it significantly impacts how we perceive and react to pain. This can make the pain feel more severe and harder to manage. For instance, the pain I experienced during dental drilling on a decayed tooth was arguably as intense, if not worse, than my migraine pain. Yet, I seemed better equipped to cope with it because my brain's higher centres were not impaired by a migraine attack at the time.

Conclusion

The brainstem, which plays a vital role in regulating essential bodily functions, becomes highly reactive during a migraine. This heightened reactivity disrupts nerve pathways, particularly those involving the 12 cranial nerves, leading to a wide range of migraine symptoms. These symptoms can persist and significantly affect a person's quality of life. The 'migraine threshold' theory sheds light on how fluctuating brain sensitivity, influenced by various factors, determines when a migraine is triggered.

Given this distinct presentation, you might assume that distinguishing migraine attacks from other common headache types would be straightforward. However, it's often far more complex. When the brainstem enters this hypersensitive state, it can mimic symptoms of various health conditions, resulting in misdiagnoses, inconclusive tests and patient frustration. Adding to the challenge, other types of headaches can closely resemble a migraine attack, making a clear and accurate diagnosis difficult in many cases.

CHAPTER 3

Migraine or Headache

Why the Confusion?

Some health issues we encounter can be incredibly frustrating. We visit the doctor hoping for a clear answer, but after receiving referrals to specialists and undergoing numerous tests and retests, our condition still doesn't fit neatly into a defined category. As a result, the path forward is far from clear.

While doctors strive to provide a clear diagnosis and a specific course of action, unfortunately, this is not always the case. Signs and symptoms of different health problems can overlap, so no matter how definite Dr Google is in giving you a diagnosis, it can be a rocky, twisted path to journey on in our pursuit of good health.

Headaches are no exception. This is particularly true for migraine, given the 80 billion individual nerve fibres packed into that 'soft drink bottle'. With so much variation between each person's brain, it's not always easy to distinguish migraine from other types of headaches to get a clear diagnosis. Yet this is important to determine the best course of action for treatment.

Confusion in Classification of Migraine

Migraine is a neurological disorder focused in the brainstem region and characterised by severe pain and disabling symptoms. In simple terms, it is defined as a headache disorder that is often one-sided, involves moderate to severe pulsating pain, and is accompanied by at least two of the following: nausea, vomiting or sensitivity to light or noise. Lasting between four and 72 hours, migraine can be triggered or worsened by physical activity.[1]

Why is it, then, that migraine is not always easy to distinguish from other headache types? Classification relies on a thorough medical history and a clear description of symptoms. You will notice headaches are not diagnosed with a specific test like most medical conditions – we use the symptoms you experience to classify your headache presentation. However, you may have found it difficult to describe what's happening during a migraine attack because your nerve pathways are so scrambled. This makes it difficult for the medical professional trying to diagnose or classify your headache into a specific type.

Adding to the complexity, there are six distinct categories of migraine, further classified into multiple variations, as shown in Table 5, which immediately increases the potential for confusion.

Table 5. Migraine Categories in ICHD-3[1]

Category	**Classification**
Migraine without aura	1 variation
Migraine with aura	14 variations
Chronic migraine	1 variation
Complications of migraine	4 variations
Probable migraine	2 variations
Episodic syndromes that may be associated with migraine	5 variations

The inclusion of the category 'probable migraine' underscores the challenges in the classification process. It applies to individuals whose headaches do not precisely fit into the standard migraine presentation but are very close. Ultimately, it becomes a subjective judgement for the specialist, albeit an informed one. 'Episodic syndromes', which occur without significant headache pain, are equally difficult to categorise. Symptoms such as nausea, vomiting, abdominal pain, vertigo or neck tightness are the primary features and can closely mimic other health conditions, making the classification process one of trial and error.

A key distinguishing feature of migraine is the intensity of pain and the accompanying symptoms.[1] If your symptoms compel you to seek refuge in a quiet, dark space rather than being able to 'push through', it is likely you are experiencing a migraine attack. Interestingly, some individuals report that the intensity of their migraine episodes can vary. In milder cases, they may still manage to function, albeit with significant limitations which can interfere with normal daily interactions. This variability often blurs the distinction between migraine and headaches, increasing the risk of misdiagnosis.

Comparing Migraine to Headache

Migraine does not always fit its classification perfectly. It relies on a subjective report from the person experiencing the attack and symptoms can be diverse and variable, even for the same individual. Consequently, migraine can sometimes resemble other headache types, such as tension-type headache (TTH).

A TTH is typically described as a pressure-like sensation on both sides of the head, with moderate pain at worst, and is only occasionally accompanied by light or noise sensitivity. Physical activity does not generally exacerbate a TTH.[1] Alternatively, when migraine pain occurs on both sides of the head (40% of the time), is of moderate intensity and non-pulsating

(50% of the time), and is accompanied by light and noise sensitivity, it could almost appear to be a TTH.

Cervicogenic headache (CGH) is another common headache type caused by pain being referred from the neck into the head. When comparing migraine to CGH, there are even more similarities. CGH is described as a one-sided headache, accompanied by neck pain (both of which are common in migraine), and can also be associated with nausea, vomiting, light or noise sensitivity.[1]

Table 6. Comparison of Headache Types

Headache Type	Pain Type	Intensity	Location	Symptoms
Migraine	Pulsating (50%)	Moderate to Severe	Unilateral (60%)	N, V, LS, NS
TTH	Not pulsating	Mild to Moderate	Bilateral	LS or N
CGH	Varies	Varies	Unilateral	N, V, LS, NS

***N** = Nausea, **V** = Vomiting, **LS** = Light Sensitivity, **NS** = Noise Sensitivity*

As you can see in Table 6, many symptoms of these three headache types are the same, which may make it difficult for doctors to accurately determine the specific type of headache a person is experiencing.

The Link Between Headache Types

The main reason many headache types exhibit similar symptoms and are challenging to classify is their link to a common nerve pathway known as the trigeminocervical nucleus (TCN), as shown in Figure 5.

Figure 5. The Trigeminocervical Nucleus (TCN)

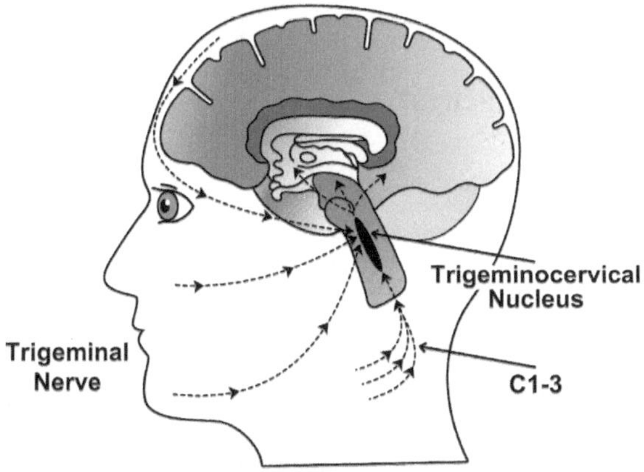

The meeting point between the trigeminal (sensory) nerve to the face and the nerves of the upper neck (C1–3).

The TCN is a meeting point for sensory (sensation) nerves that come from the face and upper head (via the trigeminal nerve) and the upper neck (C1–3). Here they connect and share information before the messages are taken up to the brain. This connection point, the TCN, sits in the brainstem, which is the highly efficient 'computer hub' that keeps your body running smoothly without conscious effort.

The TCN processes sensory signals from the upper neck and head before relaying them to the cortex for interpretation. When dysfunction arises in the upper neck, the brain may misinterpret the pain as coming from the head. This phenomenon, known as referred pain, is a defining feature of CGH and can also heighten sensitivity in the brainstem region.

As a result, migraine, TTH and CGH may all present with symptoms such as nausea, vomiting and sensitivity to light and noise. Increased sensitivity of the TCN is often present in all these headache types, thereby producing symptoms similar to a migraine. This shared mechanism is a critical factor that must be addressed in many headache presentations.[2,3]

Co-existence of Headaches

In addition to the similarity of symptoms, another reason why headache types are difficult to distinguish is they often co-exist. Having migraine disease does not exclude the possibility of also experiencing CGH or TTH. Due to these overlaps, isolating different headache types and determining a person's headache classification can be challenging.

Consider a practical example from a recent scientific report.[4] In this account a person consulted a physiotherapist with a headache that closely resembled a migraine. It is worth noting that, in my experience, someone presenting with a similar headache would often be diagnosed with migraine and prescribed medication. However, in this instance, the physiotherapist identified specific neck dysfunction. Through manual therapy and neck exercises, the physiotherapist was able to reduce the person's headaches from 16 days per month to just three days per month.

In such cases, it is possible that the person is experiencing a cervicogenic headache mimicking a migraine, or perhaps both a migraine and a cervicogenic headache occurring simultaneously. Accurately determining the type of headache, in many circumstances, may require assessment by more than one health professional – in this example, both a physiotherapist and a neurologist. In my experience, neurologists often require assistance in identifying whether the neck is contributing to a headache, as this falls outside their area of expertise.

Due to the overlapping symptoms and the co-existence of different headache types, a correct diagnosis or classification is crucial. For an individual with migraine symptoms, keeping a diary of episodes and subsequent symptoms is the best way to help health professionals determine the best course of action for treatment.

Confusion of Migraine in Youth

Diagnosing childhood migraine is another area of confusion due to its different presentation early in life. You may think that with the genetic involvement in migraine it would easily be identifiable from a young age. It is not always as obvious as you might think. Most people don't recall having migraine as a child as symptoms are not similar to migraine as we know it. A child's developing brain responds to genetic predisposition in unique ways. However, the signs are there if you know what to look for.

Migraine affects close to one in 10 children, and the likelihood of symptoms increases as they grow older. At seven years of age, the prevalence is estimated to be 1–3%, but by 15 years, it rises to 4–11%. As a child matures, migraine is more likely to become an issue.[5]

In adults, migraine is more common in females than males. It is generally estimated that 18% of females and 6% of males are affected, equating to roughly three females for every male. However, before puberty (under 11 years of age), the ratio is closer to 50:50 between females and males.[5–9]

One of the most common things clients share with me is that their migraine attacks seemingly appeared out of nowhere, often beginning in their late teens or early twenties. They are often confused when it is suggested they may have experienced migraine as a child without realising it. How could they have forgotten instances of such severe pain and dysfunction? Many react with scepticism when told they've been predisposed to migraine since birth. The late onset of symptoms can make it difficult for them to acknowledge the genetic aspect of migraine.

The severity and types of symptoms in children can vary widely, making diagnosis challenging. A child's migraine may present as vague tiredness or occasional nausea, which might simply be dismissed as 'having a bad day'. In more extreme cases, symptoms such as significant fatigue, headache and nausea or vomiting are present, making an early diagnosis more likely. As children grow older, their symptoms often become more recognisable, or they develop the ability to better describe how they feel, leading to a clearer diagnosis.

Indeed, the early warning signs of migraine can be confusing and are often misdiagnosed or overlooked. These early signs may include:

- **Colic in babies:** A parent with migraine is twice as likely to have a baby with colic, which affects one in five babies under four months. Persistent colic over a three-month period increases the likelihood of developing migraine later.[10,11]

- **Abdominal pain:** Recurrent abdominal pain without vomiting may signal early migraine. Vomiting often develops with age, and the pain resolves quickly without affecting appetite or bowel movements.

- **Neck torticollis:** Babies may hold their head to one side for long periods, with intermittent neck tightness occurring without clear cause.[7,11]

- **Poor sleep patterns:** Children with migraine often experience shorter, lower-quality sleep compared to peers.[12,13]

- **Motion sickness:** Nausea during movement is strongly linked to brain areas associated with migraine.

- **Allergic-type sinus conditions:** Hay fever or conjunctivitis, often triggered by pollen or wind, is more common in children who later develop migraine.[8,9]

The incidence of these symptoms in babies is generally high and can be triggered by various factors, not just migraine. However, if there is a family history of migraine, it's worth noting the frequency of these issues without becoming overly vigilant.

There is also significant literature suggesting that childhood migraine often begins after an 'adverse childhood experience' (ACE). These experiences can include a wide range of traumatic events that may trigger migraine episodes.[14-19] Examples include parental divorce, exposure to or experience of violence or abuse, or the loss of a loved one or pet.

My Childhood Migraine

Reflecting on my own childhood health experiences, I realise that if migraine had been better understood in the 1970s, I might have received an earlier diagnosis, leading to a more effective approach to managing the condition. As it was, my childhood abdominal migraine (as I now recognise it) went largely unnoticed, dismissed as regular episodes of '24-hour tummy bugs'. These episodes typically occurred in the morning, then settled later in the day and allowed me to eat something light, such as toast. By the next day, I would feel completely fine, which would be unusual if my body had been fighting a virus or infection.

Perhaps you, too, have memories of childhood episodes that, in hindsight, seem 'migraine-like' but felt quite different from the migraine you experience now. Although each person experiences their own unique migraine presentation, common symptoms shared by both childhood and adult migraine include head pain, fatigue, sensory sensitivity, neck pain, vertigo and nausea. However, there are consistent differences between childhood and adult migraine, as outlined in Table 7.

Table 7. Differences in Childhood vs Adult Migraine

Symptom	Childhood	Adult
Headache pain	Bilateral, frontal, described as 'throbbing' or 'pounding'. Not always present	Usually unilateral, side of head/face, described as 'pulsating'
Duration	Around 2–24 hours	Around 4–72 hours
Nausea Vomiting Abdominal pain	Often the only symptom present	Can be the only symptom but more commonly associated with a headache
Light sensitivity Noise sensitivity	Difficult for a young person to describe and must be inferred from behaviour	Usually more obvious to the adult
Fatigue Mood shifts Yawning	Often the only symptoms	Usually associated with the headache

For children who are genetically predisposed to migraine, half the challenge lies in distinguishing between common childhood ailments and symptoms that may indicate migraine.

If you suspect you have passed on migraine genes to your children or recognise the signs in other children within your family, you can download my free eBook for supporting children with migraine at www.mymigrainementor.com.au. Prioritising their quality of life, understanding what to look for can be invaluable in achieving an accurate diagnosis. This is a crucial step, not only for their physical health but also for their mental wellbeing. If left unmanaged, migraine can contribute to psychological stress, which only serves to worsen the condition.

More Confusion Related to Concussion

During the 2010s, the medical community began to recognise the significance of concussion as a health issue, both in the short and long term. As a headache practitioner, it became evident that concussion frequently leads to headaches. Headache related to concussion, known as post-traumatic headache (PTH), often closely resembles migraine in its presentation – so much so that some have coined the term post-traumatic migraine (PTM) to describe it. However, the underlying cause is quite different.

Concussion results from an acceleration–deceleration injury to the head, which stretches the nerves in the brain. This stretching event triggers a surge of electrical activity that, within hours, leads to a reduction in the brain's available energy. The energy deficit causes brain dysfunction, which typically takes around 30 days to return to normal levels.[20]

An audit of all patients presenting at our headache centres identified that approximately 50% of our clients had experienced some form of concussion or neck trauma prior to the onset of their headaches. Many didn't relate the onset of these symptoms to their previous injury. What truly captured my attention was the nature of the symptoms these clients described. While some reported only headaches, many experienced symptoms that were strikingly similar to those of migraine.

Migraine and Concussion – Almost 'Family'

A concussion can lead to a variety of issues, including injury to the upper neck caused by the whiplash effect. To cause a concussion, the head must experience a force of 70 to 120G, which is significant – especially when you consider that car airbags deploy at 60G of force. In contrast, a whiplash injury to the neck requires only 4.5G of force. This means that most concussions are likely to involve some degree of neck injury. Such neck injuries often result in CGHs, which, as previously discussed, also share symptoms similar to migraine.

When analysing these symptoms, it's easy to see the difficulty in separating migraine and concussion, based on the presentation alone, especially in the more chronic state. Although the symptoms for each condition are described with different wording in the literature, they say essentially the same thing, as can be seen by comparing the two in Table 8. Obviously, they have different origins – migraine being genetic and concussion being due to trauma – but they can co-exist. It is also possible that they have similar effects on the brain to cause similar symptoms.

Table 8. Comparing Symptoms of Migraine and Concussion[21–27]

Migraine	**Concussion**
Fatigue, feeling tired or weary	Fatigue or low energy, feeling slowed down
Difficulty in concentrating	Difficulty concentrating and remembering, confusion, 'in a fog'
Neck stiffness	Neck pain
Sensitivity to light and/or sound	Sensitivity to light and/or noise
Blurred vision/diplopia	Visual disturbances, blurred vision
Yawning, somnolence	Drowsiness
Pallor	Don't feel right
Nausea and/or vomiting	Nausea/vomiting
Dysarthria/joint pain	Not applicable
Tinnitus/hyperacusis	Sensitivity to noise
Ataxia not attributable to sensory deficit	Balance problems
Decreased level of consciousnes	Impaired consciousness
Dizziness	Dizziness
Irritability, anxiety, depression	Irritability, more emotional, sadness, nervous or anxious

Research has shown that for individuals who sustain a concussion-type injury, about 70% will see their symptoms resolve within four weeks. For approximately 30% of individuals, symptoms (including headache) persist beyond 30 days, a condition known as persistent post-concussion symptoms (PPCS). Headache is a predominant symptom of concussion, and for those whose symptoms last beyond three months, headache is present in approximately 80% of cases.[21-23] Distinguishing PPCS from migraine can be particularly challenging, as it rarely presents as a headache alone and is often accompanied by additional symptoms, similar to migraine.[22-24]

Comparing Brain Function in Migraine and Concussion

The symptoms of both migraine and concussion result from changes within the brain and how it functions. When these changes persist over an extended period, they can lead to the development of chronic sensitisation, where alterations in brain function become more deeply ingrained. Two key factors contribute to this process: the brain's capacity to adapt and its energy levels.

The Learned Response from Regular Overactivity

One thing we know about the brain is that it is highly skilled at learning new tasks. This ability is advantageous when it involves positive activities such as sports or playing a musical instrument. Repetition enables the brain to create more efficient pathways, making it progressively easier to hit a golf ball, play the correct musical note or maintain a rhythmic beat.

Ironically, this ability to learn through repetition can also work against us, reinforcing negative behaviours such as harmful habits. Unfortunately, the same principle applies to migraine.[27] With each migraine, the brain adapts through functional connectivity and plasticity, making the processes more efficient and, consequently, making it easier to trigger the next one. By the time you reach your breaking point, your brain has essentially become a 'lean, mean migraine machine' – if there's one thing it does effortlessly, it's triggering migraine!

The same principle applies to concussion. The longer the symptoms persist, the harder they can be to resolve. This is why it's crucial to actively treat both conditions rather than passively wait for improvement.

Sensitivity and Energy Levels in Your Brain

When examining the two critical factors of sensitivity and energy levels in the brain during migraine and concussion, we see some important distinctions. Under normal circumstances, the brain maintains a delicate balance between using energy to perform its functions and replenishing that energy to ensure the body continues to operate seamlessly. This is why the brain requires 20% of the total blood flow through our body, to replenish the energy efficiently.

During a migraine attack, the brain enters a cycle of hypersensitivity, which causes it to consume more energy than usual. This makes it difficult for individual cells to replenish their energy, leading to fatigue. Consequently, you often feel tired and flat during an attack. If a migraine episode lasts for a day, it typically takes another day for energy levels to return to normal. Hence the fatigue, often referred to as the 'migraine hangover', tends to last longer than the pain itself.

When migraine days become more frequent, a condition known as 'chronic migraine', energy levels in the brain may remain consistently below optimal. In this state, the brain operates on low energy levels, impairing its ability to function normally. This can significantly impact your daily life, limiting your capacity to navigate work, family and other responsibilities.

Concussion presents a similar pattern, but the recovery period is generally much longer. While recovery from a migraine episode may take one to two days, it typically takes around 30 days for the brain to restore normal energy levels following a concussion.

To understand more, read ***Exploring the Science: Shared Pathophysiology of Migraine and Concussion.***

EXPLORING THE SCIENCE

Shared Pathophysiology of Migraine and Concussion

Research reveals several overlapping issues in the brainstem and surrounding nerves that contribute to the shared symptoms of migraine and concussion. By understanding these underlying mechanisms, we can uncover potential treatment strategies.

Heightened Nerve Sensitivity

Nerves communicate through electrical impulses generated by the movement of chemicals in and out of nerve fibres (see Exploring the Science: Migraine Brain Activity, Chapter 1). When nerves become overly sensitive, this chemical activity intensifies, often described as 'leaky' nerves. In migraine, this hypersensitivity is linked to genetic predisposition and external triggers. In concussion, it results from the physical stretching of nerves caused by the traumatic event.

Disrupted Brain Connectivity

Studies reveal that the brain's ability to share information across different regions is impaired in both migraine and concussion, particularly in areas responsible for processing pain.[28,29] While the specific disruptions differ between the two conditions,[30] both lead to central sensitisation, a state of heightened nerve reactivity. This disruption can worsen symptoms and reduce the brain's ability to regulate pain effectively.

Cortical Spreading Depression (CSD)

Cortical spreading depression, a wave of brain activity followed by a period of inactivity, is a hallmark of migraine but also occurs in concussion. In migraine, CSD is part of the episode, often linked to aura or pain. In concussion, it is triggered by trauma, typically starting within minutes of the injury and potentially lasting for days or weeks, with varying effects on brain function.[29]

Inflammation and Chemical Changes

Inflammation, the body's natural response to injury or dysfunction, plays a role in both conditions. In migraine, inflammation may be triggered by the disease itself or external factors like diet. In concussion, it is caused by the forces acting on the brain during the injury.[31,32] These chemical changes in the brain's cells contribute to the symptoms experienced in both conditions.

Cerebral Blood Flow Disruptions

The brain relies on a steady supply of oxygenated blood, consuming about 20% of the body's total blood supply. Both migraine and concussion are associated with changes in cerebral blood flow which disrupt the brain's energy supply.[32,33] This disruption is a key reason why fatigue is a common symptom in both conditions. Additionally, these blood flow changes are linked to dysfunction in the autonomic nervous system.

These shared mechanisms – nerve hypersensitivity, disrupted connectivity, cortical spreading depression, inflammation and blood flow changes – either contribute to or result from central sensitisation. Together, they complicate the symptoms experienced in both migraine and concussion, highlighting the need for targeted treatment approaches.

Will a Concussion affect my Migraine?

If you have a family history of migraine or early signs of migraine, a concussion may worsen your symptoms or prolong your recovery.[34-36] This can also apply to individuals who have never experienced migraine but may have a genetic predisposition. Research shows that people with pre-existing migraine disease are more likely to experience intensified symptoms after a concussion.[34,37,38] However, it's important to remember that every concussion is unique, and effects can vary greatly from person to person.

For individuals with migraine who sustain a concussion, it is crucial to take the injury seriously. Persistent symptoms following a concussion, known as PPCS, may require short-term medication to break the symptom cycle. Additionally, specific rehabilitation approaches, such as upper neck treatment for headaches or aerobic exercise to address autonomic nervous system dysfunction, should be considered before relying on medication for relief. A concussion may aggravate migraine symptoms, requiring adjustments to medication and rehabilitation strategies to return symptoms to baseline.

When Migraine, Headache and Concussion Collide

When examining the classification of headaches, migraine and concussion, the overlap is evident and can often lead to confusion for both medical professionals and the general public. To effectively treat headache and migraine in our centres, a deeper understanding of concussion was needed. I embarked on this process by connecting with Complete Concussion Management Inc. (CCMI), an online teaching platform based in Toronto, Canada. I was immediately intrigued by the parallels between migraine and concussion. The term post-traumatic migraine (PTM) has been developed to describe a post-concussion headache which meets the classification of migraine, but it is important to realise that even though they appear very similar, the treatment goals differ significantly.

When treating a concussion injury, the primary goal is to restore the individual to full health. For someone with migraine, the aim is to return them to their baseline (or better) after the concussion, reflecting their usual migraine presentation. The use of migraine medications after a concussion should be viewed as a short-term solution to manage persistent symptoms, rather than a long-term approach to treatment. In contrast, the use of medication for individuals with significant migraine issues can play a vital role in maintaining a normal quality of life.

If you're unsure whether your headache is migraine-related or caused by a concussion, don't worry! The treatment suggestions and advice outlined in this book remain relevant. CCMI offers a wealth of information on concussion through podcasts, social media and their website.[23] They advocate for a holistic approach to concussion care, which I believed could have applications in the migraine space. Hence the treatment for both migraine and concussion could be as similar as their symptoms.

It may be helpful to revisit your family medical and headache history, even if you've done so before. If you suspect you are experiencing concussion-related symptoms or a different type of headache, avoid relying solely on medication to manage your symptoms. Instead, explore the treatment options available to you.

Conclusion

The challenge of distinguishing migraine attacks from other headache types is due to overlapping symptoms. Co-existing headache types may need to be addressed with treatment to help determine the true impact of your migraine. Understanding and managing migraine requires a comprehensive approach that goes beyond the surface symptoms, as there is a need for accurate diagnosis and personalised care.

Additionally, childhood migraine often presents differently to adults and is frequently misdiagnosed. Therefore, the importance of tailored diagnostic approaches across all age groups is essential.

Shared symptoms between concussion and migraine opens the door to exploring diverse treatment strategies, offering hope for improved outcomes. By addressing these complexities, you can work towards a clearer understanding of your condition and a more effective path to relief. Recognising that factors beyond genetics can exacerbate migraine disease will empower you to take proactive steps towards effective symptom management.

02

Chapter 4:

Migraine Misery – The Downward Spiral

Chapter 5:

Role of the Neck – An Unacknowledged Connection

Chapter 6:

Intrinsic Stress – A Silent Migraine Factor

SECTION 2

The Triggers

CHAPTER 4

Migraine Misery

The Downward Spiral

The quote 'Knowledge is power' is attributed to Francis Bacon, an English philosopher from the late 1500s. He was a pioneer of the scientific method, which remains fundamental in developing the medical treatments used to address health problems today. Thomas Jefferson, the third president of the United States, also used this quote in the early 1800s while working to establish the now extensive university system in his country. Jefferson further associated knowledge with happiness, safety and power.[1]

By now you've learnt four very important things:

- You have a genetic predisposition for migraine.
- Your brainstem is prone to oversensitivity, giving you a lower migraine threshold than the average population. This 'sensitisation' tends to spread through the brain via functional connectivity, impacting the ability of your brain to process information efficiently and effectively.
- The signs for migraine were likely present from your childhood.
- Many headache presentations look very similar, leading to confusion in how to classify them and consequently how to treat them effectively.

Take a moment to reflect on this, but don't let it weigh you down. While this knowledge may not immediately make you feel more powerful, safe or happy, there is still much to learn. What truly matters is how you choose to use the information available to you.

Discovering that you have a genetic predisposition for migraine (or any health condition) can feel discouraging, and it may be tempting to believe that poor health is inevitable. However, science reassures us that we don't need to adopt such a fatalistic outlook.

It's Not All About DNA

Your health is not determined solely by genetics, so don't be too quick to blame your parents just yet! There are other influences, within your control, that can help reduce the impact of migraine on your life.

Section 2 of this book explores environmental and lifestyle factors and evaluates their impact on brainstem and limbic system sensitivity. The ultimate goal is to understand how to manage these factors, helping you stay below your migraine threshold and reduce the likelihood of a migraine attack.

Throughout this book, I will introduce a range of treatments and interventions designed to help 'calm down' your brainstem region. If you are someone who wants to understand why these interventions work and the changes they bring about, Section 2 will provide the insights you need. It will empower you with knowledge about what you can adjust to make a meaningful difference in your daily life.

As you read this section, take note of the factors that resonate with you and could be contributing to your migraine. Recognising these factors, commonly known as triggers, is a crucial first step towards regaining control and managing your migraines effectively.

Two pivotal twin studies conducted around the turn of the century significantly advanced our understanding of the factors underlying migraine. A groundbreaking study in 1998 involved approximately 200 female twin pairs, both identical and non-identical. Among them, 154 twins were raised together from infancy, while 43 were raised apart. This classic 'nature versus nurture' study revealed that genetics accounted for 50% of a person's migraine presentation, while the other 50% was attributed to the environment in which they were raised.[2]

A similar study, conducted across six countries including Australia through the efforts of researchers at QUT, confirmed these findings.[3] It showed that migraine presentation is influenced equally by genetics and environmental factors. Over time, the environmental component was further divided into environmental and lifestyle factors.

Let's pause to emphasise this: while half of your migraine presentation is determined by genetics and largely beyond your control, the other half is influenced by lifestyle and environmental factors. This means that a significant portion of your migraine experience can be shaped by the choices you make and the way you live your life. These decisions can deeply influence how nerve pathways transmit messages within your brain. When these pathways become hypersensitive, they may lead to significant limitations in your daily life.

The good news is that by identifying and managing the lifestyle and environmental factors within your control, you can take proactive steps to minimise the impact of migraine on your wellbeing.

Genetics–Lifestyle–Environmental Interactions

The challenge in understanding the relationship between genetics, lifestyle and environmental factors in migraine lies in their interconnectedness. These elements don't function independently; instead, they influence one another, and their combined effects can amplify the impact on migraine presentation.

Think of it like baking a cake. Genetics serve as the recipe, lifestyle choices are the ingredients and environmental factors are the cooking conditions. Even if you follow the recipe perfectly and use the finest ingredients, an incorrect oven temperature or overcooking can ruin the cake. Similarly, substituting salt for sugar will result in an inedible dessert, no matter how well it's baked. If the recipe is flawed, the ingredients are poor and the cooking process is mishandled, the result will be a disaster. The more things that go wrong, the worse the outcome.

This analogy applies to migraine. The interplay between genetics, lifestyle and environmental factors can significantly influence nerve sensitivity, which in turn affects the frequency, intensity and duration of migraine episodes. While we may be born with genetic predispositions to migraine, the environment we live in and the lifestyle choices we make can exacerbate its presentation.

Lifestyle and environmental factors can further increase central sensitisation, essentially turning up the 'volume' on nerve sensitivity. In a brain that is already more sensitive than average, this heightened baseline sensitivity makes it even easier to trigger a migraine episode. For example, if your genetic baseline places you at four on the hypothetical Life Impact Graph shown in Figure 6, poor lifestyle situations or environmental circumstances could elevate that to six or seven, making migraine episodes more frequent and severe.

Figure 6. Life Impact Graph

Low impact			High impact
0	X Genetics	X Genetics and lifestyle/ environment	**10**

This interplay highlights the importance of addressing lifestyle and environmental factors to manage migraine effectively. While genetics may set the stage, the choices we make can significantly influence the outcome.

The Brainstem and Survival Mechanisms

Before delving into the significant influence of environmental and lifestyle factors on migraine, it's helpful to understand why their impact is so profound. The answer lies in the brain's primary role – to ensure safety and survival.

A critical function of the brainstem and the limbic system, shown in Figure 7, is to regulate mechanisms that help us survive and adapt to our environment. One of these mechanisms is homeostasis – the body's ability to maintain a stable internal state despite changes in the external environment. For instance, maintaining a core body temperature of 37°C is vital for survival, and the brain is constantly working behind the scenes to ensure this balance.

This primitive, nonconscious part of the brain is responsible for monitoring and regulating countless systems that keep us alive and functioning. From controlling heart rate and blood pressure, to managing hormone levels and body temperature, the brainstem and limbic system are the unsung heroes of our survival. Key components of the limbic system include the hypothalamus, thalamus, hippocampus and amygdala. The brain pathways controlling these systems must remain in balance to ensure our safety. Any disruption to this balance can have far-reaching effects on our health, including migraine presentation.

Figure 7. The Brain and Survival Mechanisms

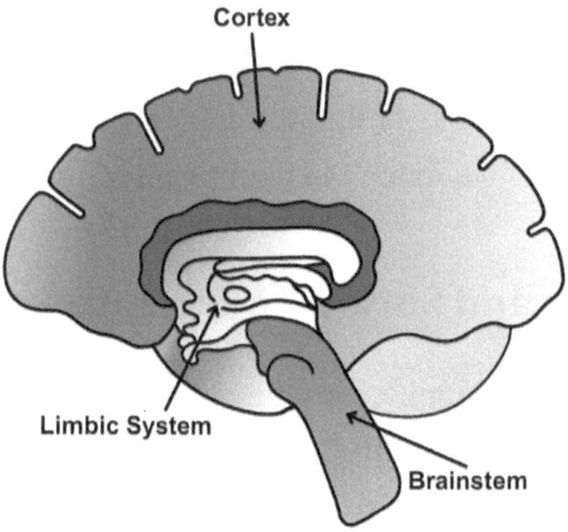

Key mechanisms in our brain controlling survival are found in the brainstem and limbic system (or the nonconscious brain).

Understanding this foundational role of the brain pathways helps us appreciate why environmental and lifestyle factors can have such a significant impact on migraine. These factors can disrupt the delicate balance the brain works so hard to maintain, increasing the likelihood of triggering a migraine episode.

When environmental and lifestyle factors place a physical or psychological 'load' on the body, it is the brainstem and hypothalamus that step in to assess the situation and make adjustments to maintain homeostasis. For example, when it's hot, the body sweats to cool down, and when it's cold, we shiver to generate heat. While these changes are controlled by the brain, their effects are visible in the body.

However, when the load becomes excessive or prolonged, the body's ability to maintain balance can falter, leading to what is often referred to as 'stress intolerance'.[4] This term describes an individual's inability to cope with the stress they are experiencing. A homeostasis system that is struggling to manage the load will often express problems through the autonomic nervous system (ANS) and the hypothalamus-pituitary-adrenal (HPA) axis. Environmental and lifestyle factors can disrupt these systems, potentially contributing to the onset or exacerbation of migraine. By addressing these factors, it may be possible to reduce the load on these systems, improving both overall wellbeing and migraine disability.

For more information on these two key systems, read ***Exploring the Science: Understanding the Roles of the ANS and HPA Axis in Stress Regulation.***

EXPLORING THE SCIENCE

Understanding the Roles of the ANS and HPA Axis in Stress Regulation

Autonomic Nervous System

The ANS is responsible for balancing two opposing states: the 'fight-flight-freeze' response, controlled by the sympathetic nervous system (SNS), and the 'rest and digest' response, managed by the parasympathetic nervous system (PNS). The SNS response is activated during stress, increasing heart rate and blood pressure, and redirecting blood flow from the gut to the muscles to prepare for action. Conversely, the PNS response promotes relaxation, digestion and recovery by directing blood flow to the gut and away from the muscles. Ideally, the body should spend most of its time in the PNS state, only activating the SNS response when absolutely necessary.

Note: *From this point on we will refer to 'fight-flight-freeze' as the SNS response and 'rest and digest' as the PNS response.*

Hypothalamus-pituitary-adrenal Axis

The HPA axis is a collection of three glands that regulate the body's response to stress by releasing cortisol into the bloodstream. Cortisol plays a crucial role in providing the energy needed to cope with stress, fuelling the body's ability to respond to immediate challenges. However, chronic activation of the HPA axis due to prolonged stress can lead to imbalances, which may manifest as physical or psychological symptoms, including migraine.

Over-Reactive Survival Mechanisms

During a migraine, the neurological pathways become over-reactive, amplifying the body's response to any physical or psychological load. This heightened sensitivity is often caused by an exaggerated reaction in key systems, such as the ANS and the HPA axis. As a result, the body struggles to maintain homeostasis, and the response to stress becomes inefficient. In the case of migraine, this inefficiency manifests as an extensive and often incapacitating bodily reaction.

This heightened response can be particularly challenging as migraine attacks often strike during the busiest and most demanding times in life, when optimal functioning is crucial. This cruel irony adds to the burden of living with migraine disease, as it disrupts daily activities and responsibilities. To better understand and manage migraine, it's essential to review the various interactions in your environment and lifestyle that may contribute to an increased migraine response.

Environmental Factors

Environmental factors refer to events or conditions largely beyond our control. Understanding how these factors influence migraine presentation is crucial, as the environments in which we live can significantly impact our health. While these factors are often uncontrollable, there are strategies that can be implemented to help mitigate their adverse effects. Key environmental factors include weather conditions, sleep quality and stressful situations.

Where You Live

When I first began treating individuals with migraine, I assumed that if there were any seasonal variations, migraines would worsen during winter. Colder weather, I thought, would likely increase physiological stress and tension, thereby elevating migraine risk. However, my interaction with patients and understanding of the research has revealed a greater complexity exists with regards to the weather and migraine.

A Japanese study conducted in 2011 found that migraine attacks were more likely to occur when air pressure dropped and less likely when air pressure rose.[5] Similarly, an American study reported that lightning increased migraine frequency by 30%.[6] Other research has also linked migraine to environmental factors such as wind, high temperatures, humid conditions and rain.

It seems that more volatile weather extremes and sudden changes seem to increase the frequency of migraine episodes. I recall treating a woman from Switzerland who reported her migraine attacks were worse during the northern hemisphere winter, particularly during snowstorms. This aligns with the idea that the migraine brain, especially the hypothalamus – responsible for thermoregulation – may overreact to extreme weather changes in an effort to maintain a stable body temperature of 37°C.

As is often the case with migraine, individual experiences vary greatly. For instance, the Japanese study found that 36% of participants reported no impact of barometric pressure changes on their migraine episodes.[5] This draws attention to the complexity of migraine and the importance of understanding each person's unique triggers and experiences.

Your Sleep Quality

Sleep is a critical lifestyle factor that can significantly influence migraine, yet it is also shaped by environmental factors and circumstances beyond our control. For instance, hot, humid nights or unsettled children can disrupt sleep patterns, which may, in turn, impact migraine presentation – either positively or negatively.

One study found that individuals who slept for shorter durations experienced higher migraine intensity and were more likely to wake with a headache.[7] In fact, 71% of participants in the study reported waking with a headache, while an intriguing 85% indicated that they would sleep, either by choice or necessity, to help alleviate the headache phase of their migraine.

The link between poor sleep patterns and migraine is well established.[8,9] Poor sleep patterns are often present in childhood migraine so the patterns can be established early in life. Sleep is partially regulated by the ANS, which makes sense given its vital role in survival mechanisms. Furthermore, the neurological and chemical pathways in the brainstem that are shared between sleep and migraine suggest that these two processes can negatively influence one another.[10] This interplay can lead to an increased migraine response, which may further degrade sleep quality over time, creating a vicious cycle.[11] Additionally, the brain's plumbing process – the glymphatic system – which drains the noxious chemicals from the brain, relies upon good sleep patterns to do its job effectively.[12] This more recent finding is another reason why inadequate sleep patterns are detrimental to a person experiencing migraine disease.

In an attempt to address sleep-related issues, people often first turn to medication, with melatonin gaining popularity in more recent times.

However, physical responses to melatonin can vary significantly. Research indicates that many melatonin supplements contain inconsistent levels of the active ingredient, which may contribute to these variable outcomes.[13]

Instead, many sleep specialists recommend natural methods to break the cycle, particularly for chronic sleep deprivation. These approaches often focus on establishing a consistent sleep routine and fostering relaxation before bedtime. By prioritising these strategies, individuals may improve both their sleep quality and their migraine management.

The Stress Impacting Your Life

Stress is undeniably a significant factor in migraine presentation, particularly when it comes to acute stress caused by major, immediate events that demand our full attention and action. These stressful events create environments that are impossible to escape, and their impact on migraine is profound.

Research has shown that an adverse childhood experience (ACE) can act as a trigger for migraine in children. If such experiences can influence migraine in youth, it stands to reason that acute stressors in adulthood will also contribute to migraine presentation.

The widespread impact of acute stress has been evident in recent years. For example, in Japan in 2018, a disastrous flooding event led to a substantial increase in the purchase of acute migraine medications.[14] Similarly, the COVID-19 pandemic has had a global psychological impact, with many individuals reporting at least one COVID-related factor contributing to an increase in migraine response.[15]

Natural disasters, such as bushfires and floods, introduce both physical and psychological stressors that further confirm the relationship between acute stress and migraine. In Australia, the 2019 bushfire season was particularly severe, lasting from September to February. In Sydney, the lingering smell of smoke for months was a constant reminder of the fires. Not only has inhaled bushfire smoke been shown to have an inflammatory effect on the brain,[16] which likely exacerbates migraine responses, but the continuous reminder of the natural disaster occurring near people's homes was a constant source of stress. This was followed by widespread flooding in the subsequent two years, compounding the stress for many individuals.

These acute stressors can overload the ANS and HPA axis, increasing sympathetic nervous system activity and, consequently, migraine responses. Understanding the role of acute stress in migraine underscores the importance of stress management strategies to mitigate its impact on overall health and wellbeing.

Lifestyle Factors

Lifestyle factors encompass various aspects of our daily lives that we have some degree of control over. Recognising how the choices you make each day can influence your migraine presentation is crucial to limiting the impact your genetics will have on your life. By consistently making informed and healthier decisions, you can positively affect your migraine brain and overall wellbeing. Key lifestyle factors include diet, stress management, exercise, hormonal fluctuations and medication use. Among these, diet seems to garner the most attention.

Diet Dominance

Most people are well aware of the critical role diet plays in maintaining overall health. This connection extends to migraine as well. It's common for individuals to focus on dietary triggers when trying to identify factors that influence their migraine attacks. This focus is partly due to the strong connection between the brain and the gut, often referred to as the gut-brain axis (GBA).

The GBA is a fascinating area of research that highlights the intricate connection between our gastrointestinal tract and brain. This bi-directional relationship means that the gut and brain can influence each other in both beneficial and harmful ways. While much of the research has focused on conditions like dementia, multiple sclerosis and epilepsy, the link between the GBA and migraine is becoming increasingly evident.

Studies suggest that migraine may be connected to gut disorders across different life stages. For instance, colic in babies has been proposed as a potential early indicator of migraine.[17] In youth, vomiting is a common symptom associated with migraine,[18,19] while in adults, conditions like irritable bowel syndrome and celiac disease have been linked to migraine.[20,21] Understanding the relationship between gut and brain health and how they influence each other is an important step in your journey.

Much of our current understanding of the GBA stems from animal studies. However, as research advances, these findings are increasingly being applied to human studies, shedding light on innovative ways to manage conditions like migraine. This expanding body of evidence underscores the critical role of gut health in a holistic approach to managing migraine and enhancing overall wellbeing.

For more information on this topic, read ***Exploring the Science: The Gut-Brain Connection in Migraine.***

EXPLORING THE SCIENCE

The Gut-Brain Connection in Migraine

The migraine brain is inherently 'wired up', meaning it is already highly sensitive. Any additional factors that further increase this sensitivity are likely to worsen migraine symptoms. Research suggests four potential mechanisms through which the gut may heighten brainstem sensitivity.

Inflammation and the Blood-Brain Barrier: An unhealthy gut can release inflammatory cells that trigger systemic inflammation, including in the brain. This inflammation can compromise the blood-brain barrier, leading to heightened nerve sensitivity in the brainstem. A poor diet often contributes to an unhealthy gut, which in turn increases nerve sensitisation and the likelihood of migraine.[21,22]

Gut Microbiome and Neurotransmitter Production: The gut microbiome plays a crucial role in producing neurotransmitters like serotonin and gamma-aminobutyric acid (GABA), which have a calming effect on the brain's 80 billion nerve cells.[23] When gut health is compromised, the production of these 'calming' neurotransmitters decreases, resulting in heightened brain sensitivity and more severe migraine responses.

Stress Response and the HPA Axis: The HPA axis, which regulates the brain's response to stress, is influenced by gut health. An unhealthy gut can intensify the stress response, as shown in animal studies, limiting the brain's ability to regulate and calm itself. This heightened stress response can further exacerbate migraine.[24]

Vagus Nerve and Brainstem Sensitisation: The vagus nerve, which serves as the primary communication pathway between the gut and brain, directly influences the brainstem. When the gut is unhealthy, the vagus nerve transmits dysfunctional signals to the brainstem, leading to increased nerve sensitisation in this region.[23,24]

These mechanisms clearly demonstrate the significant impact gut health can have on brain health. What you eat plays a vital role in maintaining a healthy gut, which in turn supports better brain function and migraine management.

The Connection Between Diet and Migraine

While much of the focus on diet and migraine revolves around identifying individual triggers, many experts now emphasise the importance of the GBA and its role in overall dietary habits. The choices we make in our diet can have profound effects on brain health, which in turn influences the severity and frequency of migraine.

Research suggests that an inadequate diet can negatively impact the brain by causing vitamin deficiencies, disrupting the gut microbiome or triggering histamine responses due to certain foods. These problematic foods are often highly processed, rich in carbohydrates, sugars and unhealthy fats. Fast foods, processed meats, alcohol and fermented products like certain cheeses are common culprits.

Histamine, a chemical that regulates sleep–wake cycles, can accumulate in excess, leading to an inflammatory response that negatively affects the brain and disrupts sleep. This inflammation can heighten brainstem sensitivity, worsening migraine symptoms.

For individuals experiencing migraine, avoiding processed and fast foods can be particularly challenging. These foods are often quick and easy to prepare, which is appealing when migraine makes day-to-day survival the priority. Breaking free from this negative dietary cycle can be one of the most significant challenges, especially for those with chronic migraine.

Dietitians working with migraine sufferers should understand that the brain has higher energy demands than usual. The brain already consumes up to 25% of the body's total energy, and for those with migraine, this demand is likely even greater. Unfortunately, the migraine brain is less efficient at utilising energy from glucose (sugars and carbohydrates) and ketones (fats). This inefficiency often leaves the brain undernourished and deficient in essential nutrients, further exacerbating migraine symptoms.

Adding to the complexity is the fact that no single diet has been scientifically proven to reduce migraine for everyone. While diets like the 'epigenetic diet' or 'gluten-free diet' may work for some, the individual nature of migraine, shaped by unique genetic factors, makes it difficult to find a universal solution.[25-27]

What Do We Know About Diet?

Despite the challenges, there are some clear principles regarding diet and migraine:

- **Avoid inflammatory foods:** Processed foods high in sugar can trigger inflammation, increasing migraine severity. While sugary foods may provide a quick energy boost, they fail to sustain the body and brain over time, leaving them undernourished. Additionally, comorbidities like heart disease or diabetes can worsen with such diets.
- **Address nutrient deficiencies:** Diets lacking essential vitamins and minerals, such as magnesium, zinc and vitamin B, can increase migraine disability. A high-sugar diet also disrupts the gut microbiome, which negatively impacts both gut and brain health.
- **Consider obesity:** While obesity is a complex issue, influenced by both physical and psychological factors, it has been linked to the

chronification of migraine. Any dietary changes that help manage weight can positively impact migraine management.[28]

Daily Stress Response

Stress related to the busyness of life is a common issue for many people living in the western world. The pressure to maintain a high work ethic and establish a comfortable lifestyle can counterintuitively create a life full of stress.

Many people work hard to provide a home and regular holidays for their family. It can take long hours of work and sacrifice to make it happen. This can create a stress-filled life with no time to relax and unwind, no time for mindfulness and meditation which helps us to de-stress. Although there is more cultural awareness of the need to have some work–life balance, it is not always easy in those middle years when a growing family and work pressures consume every available minute of your day.

After a few years of this busy lifestyle, the ANS insidiously wires up, which leads to a chronic sensitisation of the nervous system, increasing the risk of migraine episodes. This can be especially true when a person has a tendency towards anxiety, a mental health issue which can heighten the stress response.

How we respond to stress is also a significant health issue for many people. An inadequate or poor response to stress has been linked to numerous disease processes, both mental and physical. When it comes to migraine, your response to stress is recognised as a key factor. When the brain perceives a threat, the SNS is activated, initiating the 'fight-flight-freeze' response. While this reaction is a normal and necessary survival mechanism, it is designed to be short-lived. The PNS should then step in to restore balance and calm the body.

However, in circumstances where a busy lifestyle has produced chronic stress, this balance becomes disrupted, keeping the SNS in a prolonged state of overdrive. This leaves the brain in a constant wired-up state, where the sympathetic response becomes dominant.[29] This can lead to a sensitisation of the brain, particularly the brainstem region, which increases the likelihood of a migraine attack being triggered.

The impact of stress can also be amplified by the aforementioned GBA, the critical two-way communication between the gut and the brain. The connection between stress and the gut is often evident in the 'sickening' sensation many people experience during moments of stress and anxiety. Prolonged stress can lead to significant changes in gut function through both neurological pathways, such as the vagus nerve, and chemical pathways, including inflammatory responses. These changes can further exacerbate migraine symptoms, creating a vicious cycle between stress, the gut and the brain.

For more information on this topic, read ***Exploring the Science: The Interplay of Stress and Diet.***

EXPLORING THE SCIENCE

The Interplay of Stress and Diet

The two lifestyle factors – diet and stress – are deeply interconnected and play a significant role in overall health and wellbeing. While they may seem unrelated at first glance, research over the past two decades has revealed how closely they influence each other and impact various aspects of our physical and mental health.

A key connection lies in the similarities between the gut lining and the blood-brain barrier, with up to 75% of their functions being alike. This overlap explains why inflammation in one can directly impact the other. For instance, inflammatory cells affecting the brain can also disrupt gut health, creating a harmful feedback loop. An unhealthy gut exacerbates brain health issues, while a stressed brain further impairs gut function, perpetuating the cycle.

Over time, this ongoing interaction increases brainstem sensitivity, which can intensify migraine symptoms. Understanding and addressing both diet and stress is essential to breaking this cycle and supporting better overall health.[20,30,31] This intricate relationship often resembles a 'chicken-or-egg' dilemma, making it challenging to pinpoint where to begin addressing the issue. However, with the right strategies, consistent effort and patience, it is possible to interrupt this cycle and pave the way towards better health.

Exercise Effect

Exercise is recognised as part of the classification of migraine in the *International Classification of Headache Disorders, 3rd edition (ICHD-3)*. According to this classification, migraine can either be triggered by physical activity or limit one's ability to engage in exercise, particularly vigorous activities that elevate heart rate. This is thought to be linked to changes in cerebral blood flow caused by dysfunction in the ANS. However, while the classification suggests that exercise may more commonly trigger migraine episodes, this could be a misrepresentation of its overall impact.

Like sleep, exercise is a potential trigger that can also serve as a treatment when approached correctly. It is one of the most critical interventions for concussion management and could be a powerful tool for individuals living with migraine disease, as it helps address ANS dysfunction.

A recent comprehensive study conducted by a group of eight physiotherapists, a doctor and a psychologist reviewed 60 research papers on the relationship between migraine and exercise.[32] Their findings identified two types of exercise – moderate-intensity aerobic exercise and yoga – as having a high probability of delivering positive results. These exercises were shown to reduce the frequency, intensity and duration of migraine attacks while also improving overall quality of life. Other forms of exercise, such as high-intensity interval training (HIIT), continuous low-intensity exercise, Tai Chi and strength training, demonstrated a moderate probability of achieving similar benefits. This evidence strongly supports the recommendation of exercise as an effective treatment for managing migraine.

Aerobic exercise has been a cornerstone of concussion treatment for over a decade, specifically targeting ANS dysfunction. Aerobic exercise also offers indirect benefits that can positively influence migraine management, such as improved sleep, enhanced cardiovascular efficiency, reduced inflammation and better psychological wellbeing.[33,34] Additionally, it contributes to better general health outcomes, including reduced obesity and a lower risk of heart attacks and strokes – both of which are known comorbidities of migraine. The cumulative effect of these benefits, even if limited to improved sleep and ANS function, can significantly accelerate progress in managing your migraine disease.

Some researchers have even suggested that reducing obesity may enhance the effectiveness of migraine-specific medications.[35] These combined benefits make aerobic exercise one of the most appealing and impactful interventions for migraine management.

For those hesitant to engage in physical activity due to concerns about worsening migraine, research provides reassurance. One study involving 26 individuals with migraine implemented an aerobic exercise program three times a week for 12 weeks. Participants reported significant improvements in their migraine symptoms, with only one instance of exercise triggering a migraine attack.[36] This equates to just one migraine in 936 aerobic workouts, or 0.1% – a negligible risk compared to the substantial benefits.

The message is clear: physical activity is a valuable and adaptable component of any migraine management program. The type of exercise can be tailored to individual preferences and circumstances, ensuring it does not exacerbate migraine symptoms. By incorporating exercise into your routine, you can unlock a range of benefits that support both migraine management and overall wellbeing.

Hormonal Influence

It is estimated that up to 6% of all women are affected by migraine related to their menstrual cycle.[37] Often referred to as menstrual migraine, it is considered one of the most challenging types of migraine to manage effectively through any form of intervention or treatment. It can be influenced by medications for contraception, so although it is an intrinsic factor it can be affected by lifestyle choices.

According to the *ICHD-3* classification, menstrual migraine is divided into two types, with the primary criterion being that the migraine occurs within two days (before or after) of the start of menstruation, at least two out of every three months. In cases of 'pure menstrual migraine', the migraine attack occurs exclusively during this time. However, in 'menstrual-related migraine', the woman may also experience migraine attacks at other points throughout the menstrual cycle.

The underlying theory behind menstrual migraine is that hormonal changes, primarily involving oestrogen and progesterone and occurring around day one of the menstrual cycle, can sensitise the brainstem, triggering a migraine attack.[38] The oestrogen withdrawal hypothesis, first proposed in 1972, remains the most widely accepted explanation for menstrual migraine. This theory suggests that a drop in oestrogen levels in blood plasma is the most likely trigger for the menstrual migraine process.[37] Additionally, the increased sensitivity of the brainstem during this stage of the hormonal cycle,[39] potentially due to the presence of oestrogen receptors in the trigeminocervical nucleus (TCN),[37] is a well-supported concept within the scientific community.

There is also increasing evidence that when our body's hormonal system becomes dysfunctional it can be a cause of a variety of health issues, such as mental health. It is an area of migraine management that will be worthy of further investigation in the future. Consequently, treating menstrual migraine by addressing the hormonal response remains a complex challenge. There are, however, approaches that can prove helpful, which are explored in this book.

Medication Overuse

One of the key factors contributing to the development of chronic migraine is the overuse of medication during the early or 'acute' stage of the headache phase. Medication overuse is a common issue among migraine sufferers due to the intensity of symptoms. Many individuals feel unable to endure the severe pain of a migraine attack without seeking relief through medication. In fact, some people admit to taking pain relief even when it seems ineffective. This behaviour can lead to medication overuse headache (MOH), which is characterised as a chronic, dull headache occurring on more than 15 days per month, resulting from the regular use of acute pain-relief medication over a three-month period.

The medications involved in MOH are commonly simple over-the-counter analgesics, codeine-based medications and triptans (which are more targeted migraine treatments used during the early headache phase).[40] Research indicates that when MOH is suspected, structured programs to reduce medication overuse can help approximately 50% of individuals transition back to episodic migraine presentation or significantly lower the frequency of their migraine episodes.[30,41] Treatment approaches vary depending on the type of medication being overused, whether it is basic analgesics, triptans or codeine-based medications. It is crucial to undertake medication withdrawal with medical guidance, particularly for codeine-based medications, to ensure safety and effectiveness.

If you experience regular chronic headaches and migraine, reducing your reliance on acute medication may not only decrease the frequency of your migraine attacks but also improve your overall gut health – a commonly overlooked benefit.

What About Triggers?

After exploring the various environmental and lifestyle factors that can influence brainstem sensitivity and, consequently, your migraine episodes, you may be wondering where triggers fit into this discussion. Let's delve deeper to provide some clarity and context to the role of triggers in managing migraine.

When discussing migraine, both sufferers and medical professionals often focus on 'triggers' – factors that set off a migraine attack. Recent research has explored the overlap between potential triggers and the lifestyle-environmental factors we've been discussing, proposing that a trigger could be defined as any factor that, alone or in combination with others, contributes to the initiation of a migraine.[42] Interestingly, these triggers can occur up to three days before the headache phase begins.

Identifying your triggers, however, is not as straightforward as it may seem. One study found that participants correctly identified potential triggers only 16% of the time,[43] suggesting that a more structured framework for trigger identification could be highly beneficial.

One challenge lies in the premonitory phase of migraine, which includes subtle symptoms such as fatigue or hunger. These symptoms can be misinterpreted as triggers, leading individuals to believe that hunger, or a response to something they ate, caused the migraine. In reality, these early migraine changes may be the root cause of the hunger itself.

This complex issue was addressed in a study that examined potential triggers while accounting for premonitory symptoms. Over a 90-day period, 326 participants tracked 33 potential triggers daily, including dietary, lifestyle, environmental and intrinsic factors such as neck pain and hormonal changes. The findings were revealing: 87% of participants displayed a clear trigger profile, and 84% of these profiles were unique to the individual, underscoring the highly personalised nature of migraine triggers. On average, participants identified four triggers, with some reporting over ten.[44]

The most common trigger was neck pain (43%), followed by tiredness and air temperature (both 33%). Other frequently reported triggers included restless sleep, smells/odours, bright lights, and loud noises (mid-20% range). Interestingly, some widely believed triggers, such as physical activity and certain foods (e.g. alcohol, chocolate, cheese), were reported by only 2–4% of participants.

What stands out is the overlap between migraine triggers and cranial nerve-related symptoms. For instance, environmental triggers like bright lights, loud noises and smells are processed by cranial nerves #2, #8 and #1, respectively. Food and alcohol triggers may influence cranial nerve #10, also known as the vagus nerve. Other triggers, such as stress, poor sleep, dehydration, missed meals, tiredness and weather changes, likely affect the brainstem and hypothalamus directly. These triggers appear to have a strong connection to sensory activity in the lower brain regions, which are often implicated in initiating migraine attacks.

My perspective is that sensory input from cranial nerves feed into the brainstem and lower brain regions, which, as we've discussed, is the 'migraine hotspot'. This activity can sometimes 'fire up' these regions, contributing to a migraine episode. Some argue that the process may have already begun, the migraine was inevitable, but this is difficult to prove. What is clear, however, is the significant overlap between migraine symptoms and triggers.

The research also highlights that migraine attacks are rarely caused by a single trigger.[43] Most participants required multiple triggers – on average, four – to cross the migraine threshold and initiate an attack. This challenges the common misconception that migraine is caused by just 'one thing'. Instead, it's often the combination of triggers that pushes the brain into a migraine episode.

Referring again to the Migraine Threshold Graph in Figure 8 below, it is more accurate to represent it in this manner.

Figure 8. Migraine Threshold Graph

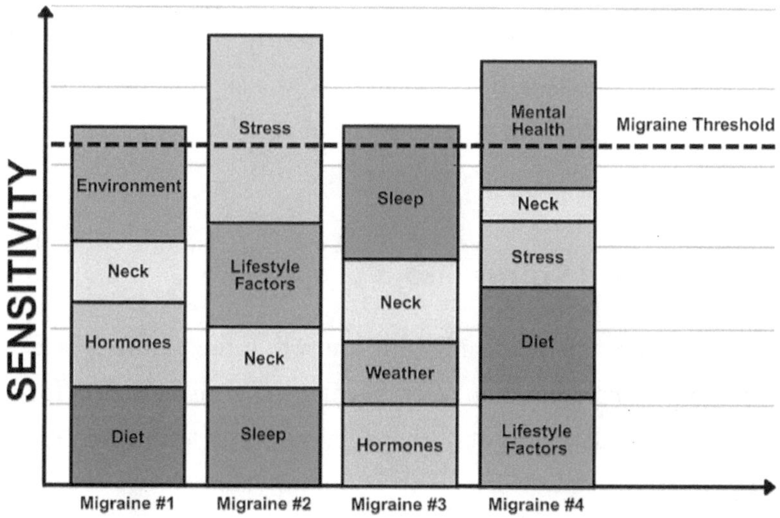

A combination of factors contribute to pushing an individual over their migraine threshold.

Most people will have a number of factors that could push their nerve sensitivity to a point where it reaches the migraine threshold and triggers a migraine attack. The same person could have different triggers for different migraine attacks, which could mean each migraine episode will present differently in intensity, duration or symptom presentation.

Many factors can contribute to the onset of a migraine attack. On one day, stress might act as the primary trigger, while on another, lack of sleep could push you over the migraine threshold. It's important to understand that migraine episodes are often the result of multiple overlapping factors. This complexity is why the trigger study required an extensive 90-day assessment to identify potential triggers. Triggers and lifestyle factors frequently overlap; what causes a migraine one day might only contribute to it on another. Yet, we often focus on the most recent factor leading to a migraine, labelling it as 'the trigger'.

When multiple factors or triggers consistently work together to push us over the migraine threshold, it can lead to a significant worsening of symptoms or an increase in the frequency of attacks, often starting a cycle that can severely impact your quality of life.

The Downward Spiral

Most people who experience migraine know that their journey is far from smooth. Migraine presentation often fluctuates over time. Reflect for a moment: can you recall a time, or perhaps several times, when your migraine attacks were noticeably worse? This is due to your survival mechanisms over-reacting.

As we navigate the winding path of life, lifestyle and environmental factors accumulate, creating conditions that can turn the road beneath us into a rocky, twisted path. This often happens, though not exclusively, around the 30- to 40-year mark.[45] It's a time when occupational stress (building a career) and family responsibilities (raising children, caring for ageing parents) converge with the lifestyle choices made up until this point – perhaps a poor diet, lack of exercise or even the environment you live in. These factors combine to create a physical response in your body, cranking up brainstem sensitivity and more frequently pushing you over the migraine threshold. This occurs because the survival mechanisms of your nonconscious brain struggle to cope with the mounting load.

I call this perfect storm of conditions 'the downward spiral'. When migraine strikes hard during these middle years, it can have a devastating impact on your ability to engage with family and loved ones,[46] often leading to further psychological stress. This has been my personal experience, as well as the experience of many patients I've worked with over the years.

It's important to acknowledge how challenging this part of the journey can be. Escaping the downward spiral takes time, patience and resilience – all of which are difficult to muster when the path beneath your feet feels like a slippery slope.

My Personal Migraine Downward Spiral

Reflecting on my migraine journey over the years, I can trace a clear progression that mirrors the challenges and changes in my life.

In childhood, I experienced regular bouts of nausea and vomiting, constant signs of light sensitivity and frequent motion sickness. These symptoms were all tied to my genetic profile and were an early indication of what was to come. As I moved into my late teenage years, the episodes of nausea and vomiting began to subside but were still occasionally triggered by lifestyle factors, such as alcohol or certain foods.

By the time I turned 30, I experienced my first severe migraine attack. It was the early 1990s, and the attack began with a persistent episode of neck pain that I had endured throughout a long day at work. On the drive home the nausea began. Upon walking into the house, I immediately vomited before collapsing into bed with a severe headache and overwhelming nausea. This marked the beginning of a more intense phase of my migraine journey.

The 1990s were a particularly demanding period in my life. I launched a physiotherapy business, managed a young family, built a house and was deeply involved with the Sydney Blues baseball team and my church community. By the late 1990s, the frequency of my migraine episodes had noticeably increased, reflecting the mounting pressures and responsibilities I was juggling.

The year 2000 brought two significant events that caused my migraine attacks to escalate further. Episodes became more frequent, occurring every four to six weeks on average, and more disabling. The intensity of the vomiting also increased, occurring every 20 minutes for six to eight hours. On two occasions, the severity of the vomiting led to hospital visits due to dehydration. It was during one of these visits that migraine was first suggested as a possible diagnosis.

From that point on, my migraine was managed with anti-nausea medication and rest. This approach continued until November 2008, marking a long and challenging chapter in my migraine journey.

You are not alone in your migraine diagnosis. Migraine affects an estimated one billion people worldwide and is the second leading cause of disability globally.[45] These statistics are staggering, but the real impact is felt in individual stories – especially if you've lived through a downward spiral yourself.

The good news is that, while this journey is challenging, it is possible to nudge your way back to more level ground. By altering certain aspects of your environment and lifestyle, you can lower your baseline nerve sensitivity, making it harder to reach your migraine threshold. In other words, you can raise your migraine threshold, reducing the likelihood of an attack. While not all factors are within your control, identifying and addressing those you can influence can make a significant difference, helping you navigate a more balanced path.

In essence, our goal is to address the factors in our lives that heighten the sensitivity of our brainstem nerve pathways. Interestingly, one of the proposed mechanisms for achieving this improvement ties back to our genetics.

While changes such as reducing medication overuse or improving gut health can significantly influence migraine, pinpointing the exact underlying cause of these improvements can be more complex. Research suggests that these changes may exert their effects through an impact on our unique genome or genetic predispositions, emphasising the intricate relationship between lifestyle factors and our genetic makeup.

Can These Factors Impact Your Genetics?

It is possible that environmental and lifestyle factors can impact a person's migraine response in ways we don't understand yet. Epigenetics is one way that is being researched widely.

You may remember from Chapter 1 that there are 44 genetic factors associated with migraine. Dr Rob Smith from QUT also pointed out that there are many genes, possibly into the hundreds, that seem to be able to influence the genes that have a direct impact on your migraine presentation.[47] This widens the possible influence of genetics on migraine but remains in the sphere of influence of our individual lifestyle choices. Consequently, what we can influence (lifestyle and environment) can impact migraine in two ways – either by direct influence on the nervous system or by a process called 'epigenetics'.

Epigenetics examines how lifestyle changes can modify the way our genes are expressed. While the DNA sequence itself remains unchanged, certain genes can be suppressed, preventing them from negatively affecting our health. This means that environmental and lifestyle factors can influence problematic genes, altering how they function in producing proteins.

Think of your genetic profile as a set of light switches in a room. While you can't change the wiring (your DNA), you can control which switches are turned on or off. Epigenetics is like the hand that flips these switches, influenced by your lifestyle choices. By adopting healthier habits, such as improving your diet and incorporating regular exercise, you can turn off the switches linked to migraine triggers and turn on those that promote better health. As a result, the frequency, intensity, duration and even the associated symptoms of migraine may be reduced. This highlights the potential for lifestyle choices to directly influence genetic activity, offering a powerful tool for managing migraine and helping you move closer to a healthier, pain-free future.

The takeaway? Making positive lifestyle changes can have a profound, multi-faceted impact on your brain and overall health. These changes not only help reduce migraine disability but also create a ripple effect of benefits, reinforcing the importance of taking control of the factors within your reach.

Conclusion

You may be starting to see why a single form of treatment isn't always effective when managing life with migraine. Even if you discover something that works, its effects may only be temporary before the migraine returns. This is often (though not always) tied to the daily choices we make – those pivotal moments where we stand at a fork in the road. The key is to consistently choose the better path over time. To do this effectively, understanding all possible pathways is essential. That's why the next two chapters are so important – they provide you with extra knowledge and tools to help you navigate your migraine journey more effectively.

In these chapters, we'll explore two often-overlooked factors in the migraine world: the upper neck and psychological stress. These elements play a significant role in migraine management, and understanding their impact could be a game-changer in your journey towards better health.

CHAPTER 5

Role of the Neck

An Unacknowledged Connection

As you deepen your understanding of migraine, I hope you begin to see a clearer path towards a happier, more fulfilling life. Knowledge has the power to drive meaningful change, but it often requires stepping outside the comfort of familiar beliefs. Challenging long-held assumptions and shifting your perspective can feel unsettling, especially when it comes to recognising the critical role the neck can play in migraine management.

Over the past 15 years, I've worked with countless migraine patients who feel frustrated – frustrated by their health, the limitations migraine imposes on their lives and families, and the lack of clarity about what's happening in their bodies. One of the most common and unnecessary frustrations I hear is when patients tell their doctor or health professional that they believe their neck is contributing to their migraine presentation, only to be dismissed and told that this isn't possible.

I respectfully disagree.

I strongly believe that the neck can play a significant role in triggering the migraine process. Consider this: in cases of cervicogenic headache (CGH), symptoms often overlap with those of migraine, such as nausea, vomiting and sensitivity to light and noise. This overlap suggests that the neck may contribute to brainstem sensitisation, a critical factor in the development of migraine. Given this connection, it stands to reason that dysfunction in the neck could similarly play a role in sensitising the brainstem, potentially contributing to the onset or exacerbation of migraine.

A recent study involving nearly 15,000 people who experience migraine across six western, first-world countries found that 70% reported neck pain as part of their migraine experience.[1] Even more striking, those with neck pain were nearly twice as likely to experience moderate to severe disability, higher rates of anxiety and depression, and significantly reduced productivity at work. They also responded less effectively to acute migraine medications. These findings underscore the profound impact the neck can have on migraine disease and disability. Importantly, addressing neck dysfunction offers an opportunity for significant physical and psychological improvement with minimal disruption to a person's lifestyle. Many physiotherapists and allied health professionals agree – a neck that isn't functioning properly can often contribute to headaches.

So why are patients still being told by some specialists that their neck couldn't be a factor in their migraine disease? The issue lies in how different disciplines interpret the research. The prevailing view is that neck pain or stiffness is merely a premonitory symptom – the first stage of the migraine process.[2] As a result, neck pain is often dismissed as a byproduct of the migraine, with the assumption that treating the migraine with medication will resolve the neck pain. However, emerging evidence suggests that neck dysfunction may actually contribute to brainstem sensitivity, potentially pushing individuals closer to their migraine threshold.

The Neck: Symptom or Trigger?

A recent study involving hundreds of individuals experiencing migraine revealed that the presentation of migraine attacks can change significantly over a five-year period.[3] The researchers concluded that numerous modifiers and modulators likely influence these changes. One such modifier could be the neck, particularly if it has been affected by an injury, such as whiplash or concussion. Additionally, modern lifestyle factors, such as prolonged periods of screen time, may also contribute to these changes.

Here's what we have currently outlined so far about the neck's connection to migraine presentation:

- We know that neck pain is a significant public health concern, particularly in developed countries and among middle-aged men and women – the demographic most affected by migraine.[4] This is not surprising to physiotherapists, who frequently treat patients with neck pain as part of their daily practice.

- We know that neck torticollis, a sustained one-sided head tilt, has been strongly associated with migraine in children.[5] In fact, a group of experts has even suggested that it should be included in the ICHD-3 classification as part of the 'migraine syndrome'.[6] Similarly, neck pain is commonly reported in adolescents with migraine, particularly among those experiencing a higher frequency of attacks.[7,8]

- We know that the neck is considered a trigger by 43% of people with migraine, making it the most commonly reported trigger – 10% higher than the next most common factor.[2] Research also shows that neck pain is closely linked to the increasing frequency or 'chronification' of migraine attacks.[1,9,10] For instance, neck pain is present in 40% of individuals with infrequent migraine attacks but rises to 70% in those with more frequent attacks.[1,10] This increase in neck pain is also associated with higher levels of disability.[1]

This evidence suggests that the neck is inextricably linked with migraine. When neck pain is present, all aspects of a person's migraine experience tend to worsen. Could it be that the neck plays a role in influencing brainstem sensitisation? Let's explore the potential impact the neck may have on the brainstem and other nonconscious areas of the brain.

Neck Connections to the Brain

A friend and colleague, Roger O'Toole, founder of Melbourne Headache Centre, has conducted extensive research into the nerve connections between the neck and the brain. By analysing the neuroscience, he has explored the potential links and influences the neck may have on the brainstem and other nonconscious areas of the lower brain. His findings reveal significant connections between the upper neck and these critical regions.

We've previously discussed how nerves from the upper neck connect to the brainstem via the trigeminocervical nucleus (TCN).

Another key area of the upper neck involves three small but vital muscles, collectively known as the occipital triangle, which also have profound connections to the brainstem.

Let's delve deeper into both the TCN and the occipital triangle, and their potential role in influencing sensitivity.

The Trigeminocervical Nucleus (TCN)

The upper neck, specifically the top three vertebrae (C1, C2 and C3) and their associated nerves, has a direct connection to the trigeminal nerve through the TCN, shown in Figure 9. This connection extends further to the vagus nerve, which influences the gut and stomach, particularly the areas responsible for nausea and vomiting. It's not uncommon for mobilisation or pressure applied to the upper neck to induce nausea in some individuals.

Additionally, the C1 nerve has connections to the hypothalamus,[11] a part of the limbic system that plays a role in the early stages of migraine generation. These intricate connections reveal the upper neck's potential to influence various brain regions involved in migraine processes.

Figure 9. The Trigeminocervical Nucleus and Connections

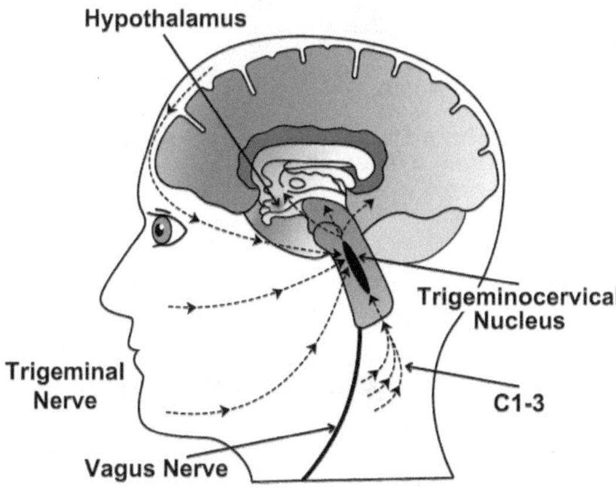

Nerves from the TCN connect with regions including the vagus nerve and the hypothalamus.

The Occipital Triangle

Another critical connection involves three small muscles that link the top three vertebrae to the base of the skull. These muscles – rectus capitis, inferior oblique and superior oblique – are collectively referred to as the occipital triangle. The nerves from these muscles also travel up through the brainstem as they transmit information to the brain, shown in Figure 10.

Figure 10. The Occipital Triangle

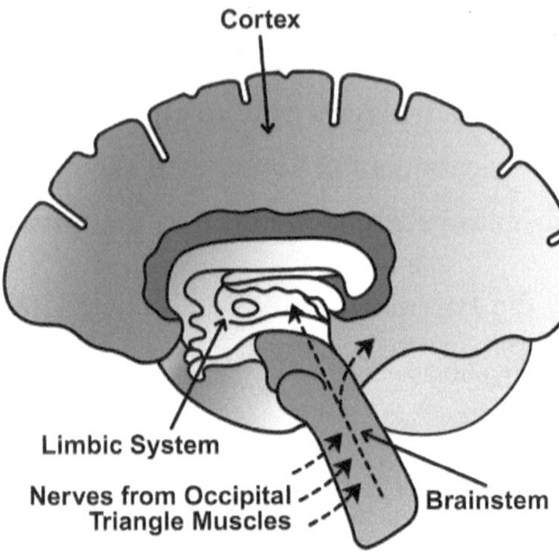

Nerves from the occipital triangle travel through the brainstem.

Despite their small size, these muscles are densely packed with receptors that monitor muscle tension. This makes them essential for transmitting neck tension information to the brainstem, particularly to areas responsible for eye movement and the vestibular system, which maintains balance and equilibrium. Furthermore, these muscles have connections to higher regions of the limbic system, which can influence the autonomic nervous system (ANS). Dysfunction in these muscles can disrupt the processing of information in these control centres, potentially contributing to symptoms similar to those experienced in migraine, such as dizziness or imbalance.

A Direct Route to Sensitivity

Both the upper neck structures – the top three vertebrae and the occipital triangle – provide significant inputs to the brainstem and limbic system. This suggests that the upper neck has the necessary neurological connections to influence these nonconscious control regions and thus sensitise the brainstem.

O'Toole hypothesises that inappropriate feedback from these most sensitive muscles in the body (occipital triangle muscles) can occur if the upper neck is not functioning properly. Due to the neurological connections and pathways in the brain this creates a significant stress, which can then activate a heightened brainstem and limbic system stress response. The brain reacts by activating the autonomic nervous system (ANS), resulting in hypersensitivity to what should be normal sensory stimulation. This is exactly the same scenario that was addressed in Chapter 4. It makes sense, too, that the neck should be hardwired into the survival mechanisms of the brainstem – we can live without an arm or a leg as the result of an accident, but we definitely need our head on our shoulders to survive. Consequently, the ANS, which governs the body's sympathetic response and overlaps with emotional responses to pain, can be influenced by a person's neck if it isn't functioning normally.

For individuals with a genetic predisposition to brainstem sensitisation, the integration of information from the upper neck vertebrae and associated nerves could contribute to this process. This may result not only in cervicogenic headaches but also in migraine attacks. Considering the connections of both the TCN and the occipital triangle, it appears that the upper neck has the potential to influence migraine through brainstem sensitisation and ANS disruption. Research into the effects of upper neck treatment on the ANS indicates that it may indeed have an influence on reducing this negative response.

Proving that upper neck dysfunction increases brainstem sensitivity is challenging, but the idea of reducing sensitivity through treatment is promising. If treating the upper neck can lower sensitivity, it suggests that dysfunction in this area might increase it. This emphasises the need to explore the upper neck's role in migraine and its potential as a treatment target.

Understanding Neck Dysfunction

To fully understand the potential impact of upper neck dysfunction, it's important to first define what 'dysfunction' actually means. For physiotherapists, neck dysfunction is not solely about pain – it encompasses a variety of factors. Modern research into how the neck functions uses a broad range of assessments, including evaluations of range of motion, strength, neuromuscular balance and control, proprioception, stability, structural issues and palpation techniques.[12-15] These comprehensive methods provide a detailed understanding of any deficits in the upper neck and, more importantly, offer strategies to address them effectively.

The important point is that the absence of neck pain does not necessarily mean your neck is functioning properly. You may unknowingly be moving your neck in an unusual pattern as your brain attempts to avoid movements that could cause discomfort. Our brains are remarkably adept at compensating for potential pain, often leading us to adjust our movements – such as turning our shoulders instead of our neck – without even realising it.

While neurologists often focus on structural changes, such as arthritis visible on CT scans or X-rays, these changes typically appear later in life and are not the sole indicators of dysfunction. Physiotherapists, on the other hand, consider these structural changes but also focus on identifying and improving other factors that influence how the neck moves and functions. This holistic approach ensures a more comprehensive understanding and treatment of neck dysfunction.

My Journey with a Problematic Neck

In my 40s, I found myself in a downward spiral with migraine. Following an episode of viral meningitis in 2000, my neck pain became worse and led to a distressingly predictable pattern. Mornings often began with a sharp, knife-like pain in my upper neck, right at the base of the skull, usually on the right side. Many of my patients describe experiencing a similar pattern. If I didn't manage to settle the pain early, it would evolve – the stabbing sensation in my neck would fade, only to be replaced by a global, throbbing head pain accompanied by disorientation. Before long, I would find myself locked into a relentless 20-minute cycle of vomiting.

One morning stands out vividly in my memory. In an attempt to relieve the pain, I pressed on my neck, only to trigger a migraine attack almost instantly. This experience reinforced my belief that my neck was a key part of the problem, even though my X-rays were clear. No one had ever told me otherwise. When I learned about a course titled "The Role of C0-C3 Segmental Dysfunction in Primary Headache – Level 1 Foundation" by Adelaide-based physiotherapist Dean Watson, I was intrigued.

Dean Watson had dedicated his career to understanding headaches. With a curious and methodical approach, he developed what is now known as the Watson Headache® Approach (WHA). This strategy focuses on assessing and treating upper neck dysfunction as a potential cause of headaches. Watson's method involves a specific assessment process using gentle mobilisation techniques to identify whether the upper neck is contributing to headache disorders. He later pursued a PhD to further explore the impact of upper neck dysfunction on headache sufferers, including those with migraine.

In late November 2008, I attended Watson's course. Over three days, I gained insights that would profoundly change my life. Thankfully, a migraine episode didn't disrupt the experience. The course provided an excellent overview of headaches and the potential role of the upper neck in their development. It was a turning point in understanding my own condition and how to help others.

The Science of the Watson Headache Approach

A defining feature of the WHA is the application of gentle pressure to specific levels of the upper neck to determine whether it reproduces a patient's 'familiar headache pain'.[16] While this may sound like a modest procedure, it can be a confronting experience for the patient. I recall treating an Irish patient who suffered from migraine centred around her right eye and temple. After explaining the concept of reproducing familiar headache symptoms, I applied light pressure to her right C2 vertebra. Her immediate response was an emphatic F-bomb, delivered in that charming Irish lilt that somehow softened the expletive. We both laughed, but the message was clear – I had successfully reproduced her familiar headache pain. This reproduction of pain is a cornerstone of the WHA and has been scientifically validated through Watson's PhD research, which measured its impact using the blink reflex.

The blink reflex, our ability to blink, is a protective mechanism that shields the eye from potential harm. In research, it can be stimulated by a small electrical pulse above the eye socket. This impulse travels through the brainstem, and the speed of the reflex can be measured to assess brainstem sensitivity – a key factor in migraine. The blink reflex has been widely used in research to evaluate the effectiveness of migraine medications on brainstem sensitivity[17–20] and is considered a reliable tool for measuring improvements. However, its use in clinical settings is limited due to the time required for set-up, the discomfort of the procedure and the complexity of analysing results.

Watson's 2014 study,[21] published in *Headache*, demonstrated that his techniques – reproducing and resolving familiar headache pain – produced an immediate reduction in brainstem sensitivity as measured by the blink reflex. More recently, similar findings were reported in the *Journal of Manual & Manipulative Therapy*, although the treatment in that study did not involve reproducing headache pain.[22] This research confirmed that mobilisation of the upper neck can reduce brainstem sensitivity, highlighting its potential as a treatment for migraine. Over the past five years, a growing body of research has linked upper neck treatment to migraine relief,[23-41] with numerous studies supporting its effectiveness.

The research is clear: mobilisation of the upper neck has the ability to reduce brainstem sensitivity. Consequently, it seems plausible to assume that upper neck dysfunction could increase brainstem sensitivity, making its involvement in migraine a distinct possibility.

Despite these developments in our knowledge, there is still much to explore. For instance, many patients report that their migraine medications seem to work more effectively after undergoing WHA treatment. If this observation is scientifically validated, it could significantly improve the quality of life for migraine sufferers.

In my experience it is also important to address other elements of neck dysfunction including muscle strength and neuromuscular control of the upper neck muscles. This will require further research to scientifically prove their importance in the treatment of migraine.

The practice of reproducing familiar headache pain during treatment has been a point of contention over the years. Some therapists question its validity, while prospective patients often worry that it might trigger a migraine attack – a reasonable psychological concern given their goal is to avoid such episodes.

To address these concerns, I offer two reassurances:

- Over the years, the WHA has evolved into a gentler technique. In the past, physiotherapy often involved forceful methods, a remnant of the 1990s. Today, we recognise that migraine involves a neurologically sensitive system, and treatment intensity is adjusted accordingly. The focus is on addressing nerve sensitivity rather than solely treating a mechanical issue in the neck.

- While the process of reproducing familiar symptoms may seem confronting, many patients find it reassuring. It validates their experience and provides a sense of understanding that they may not have encountered before. This approach not only addresses the physical aspects of migraine but may also tap into the psychological factors contributing to the condition.

Further research will help refine our understanding of the most effective upper neck treatment for migraine. The WHA continues to offer a promising, evidence-based approach that addresses both the physical and psychological dimensions of this complex condition.

Desensitising the Brainstem Through Manual Therapy

It is essential to recognise that treating migraine is fundamentally a neurological issue, not merely a mechanical problem in the neck. The goal of treating the neck is to influence brainstem sensitivity, not to aggravate the neck pain or headaches. This is why the WHA has evolved into a more refined and subtle technique. The focus is on calming the neurological system rather than aggravating it. Many patients describe the reproduction of their headache pain during treatment as a "good pain", often reporting a relieving or soothing effect. It feels as though the treatment is calming the headache rather than exacerbating it.

My Introduction to the WHA

The connection between the upper neck and migraine became evident to me early in my journey as a physiotherapist focusing in headache treatment. Shortly after completing the Level 1 Foundation course for the WHA during an intensive three-day weekend, I returned to work on Monday with a wealth of new knowledge still fresh in my mind. It wasn't long before I had the opportunity to put this knowledge into practise.

A family friend had a visitor from New Zealand who had suffered a significant head and neck injury approximately 18 months earlier. Since the injury, he had been experiencing severe, migraine-like headaches on a daily basis. When asked, "Do you

> *think you can help him?" – a question I had encountered many times as a physiotherapist – I found myself uncertain but willing to try.*
>
> *I assessed Rowan[3] and applied a basic WHA treatment, hoping for a positive outcome. To my surprise, he reported a noticeable improvement in his condition for three days before his symptoms returned to their usual pattern. Observing even a temporary change in a chronic condition like Rowan's was a pivotal moment for me. It reinforced the idea that the upper neck could play a significant role in influencing migraine presentations, making it an area worth exploring further.*

Over time I have developed the professional opinion that assessing the upper neck should be a standard consideration in any migraine presentation. This assessment can help identify specific central sensitisation of the neurological system or the coexistence of other headache types. It is important to remember that every migraine journey is unique, and an evaluation of the upper neck should always be an option for those experiencing migraine.

Dean Watson was a pioneering voice in advocating for this approach over 30 years ago, often standing alone in his perspective. Today, his methods are widely recognised and supported by many in the field, reflecting the growing understanding of the role the upper neck plays in migraine management.

---

3 Rowan is a patient (name changed for privacy) who provided consent for his story to be shared.

Developing a Team to Help Those with Migraine

I recognise the growing acceptance within the specialist neurology community in Australia of the role the upper neck plays in headaches, including migraine. Since 2019, I have been collaborating with a group of neurologists in Sydney, focusing on treating the neck component for many of their patients experiencing headaches. This association began when Associate Professor Raymond Schwartz, founding partner of Southern Neurology, reached out with the innovative idea of integrating neck treatment into their approach. This initiative has led to an effective collaboration, benefiting many of our shared patients.

More broadly, it is becoming increasingly evident that neurologists are acknowledging the influence of the complex variables we have discussed throughout this book. This shift is subtly changing the way migraine is being treated in Australia. Gradually, the two professions – neurology and physiotherapy – are beginning to align in their understanding and approach, fostering a more collaborative and holistic treatment landscape.

Conclusion

If you've been told that your neck isn't contributing to your migraine presentation and, as a result, haven't included it as part of your treatment plan, it may be time to reconsider. Similarly, if you've been receiving treatment for your neck but the approach hasn't focused on desensitisation or improving functional abilities such as strength and muscle control, it might be worth re-evaluating your strategy.

In today's screen-dominated world, neck dysfunction has become a prevalent issue. The fact that upper neck treatment can often deliver immediate and noticeable change is both encouraging and empowering for patients and therapists alike.

Scientific literature increasingly recognises that 'sensitisation' is not just a physical response but a holistic one, shaped by the interaction of physical, psychological and social factors.[42] Each person's pain response is influenced by their unique traits and the environment surrounding their headache experience.

However, before embarking on the journey to improvement, it's essential to address the psychological factors at play. Psychological stress is a significant contributor to migraine, and when combined with other life pressures, it can trap individuals in a persistent stress response. Understanding and managing these psychological factors is a crucial step in breaking free from this cycle and paving the way for sustainable improvement.

CHAPTER 6

Intrinsic Stress

A Silent Migraine Factor

It has long been recognised that our response to stress is intricately linked to migraine, although early psychological analysis missed the mark. You may recall that in the 1970s, migraine was mistakenly classified as a psychiatric disorder, often associated with unfounded and stigmatising assumptions about psychotic behaviour. Thankfully, as our understanding of migraine has evolved, so too has our awareness of the complex and symbiotic relationship between stress, migraine and psychological health.

This growing body of knowledge has undoubtedly improved the treatment of migraine, fostering approaches that enhance the overall wellbeing and quality of life for those affected. By addressing both the physical and psychological dimensions of migraine, these advancements have helped many individuals find a safer and more fulfilling space in the world. However, the journey of living with migraine disease remains a challenging one, as the stress associated with this condition continues to weigh heavily on those who experience it.

Even as far back as the 1970s, the role of the autonomic nervous system (ANS) in migraine was acknowledged. A 1973 study explored the influence of personality traits and stressful experiences on migraine, revealing that events which heightened sympathetic nervous system (SNS) activity were involved in over 50% of migraine attacks.[1] While migraine is no longer viewed as a psychiatric defect or mental illness, it is clear that negative psychological experiences can act as powerful triggers. Most migraine sufferers are all too familiar with how stress – whether from work, home or other life pressures – can set the stage for an episode to begin.

Extrinsic and Intrinsic Stress

We've already explored how chronic lifestyle stress can accumulate and heighten brainstem sensitivity through mechanisms like the ANS and the hypothalamus-pituitary-adrenal (HPA) axis, ultimately worsening migraine symptoms. Similarly, we've discussed how acute stress – such as adverse childhood experiences (ACEs) – can trigger the onset of migraine in children. These forms of stress are often referred to as 'extrinsic' stress, as they stem from external factors which may or may not be under the individual's control.

For many people living with migraine, however, there is an additional layer of stress that is ever-present: the constant fear of an attack striking at any moment. This ongoing burden influences daily decisions, strains relationships with loved ones and casts a shadow over every aspect of life. This type of stress, which arises internally, can be described as 'intrinsic'. Unlike extrinsic stress, intrinsic stress is deeply personal and often invisible to others.

The hidden nature of intrinsic stress makes it especially insidious. It often goes unnoticed by friends, family and colleagues, and even the individual experiencing it may fail to recognise its gradual onset. Its slow and subtle build-up can make it difficult to identify until it has already taken a toll. Yet, intrinsic stress compounds the effects of extrinsic stress, further amplifying the SNS response and exacerbating the cycle of migraine.

The critical role of stress in migraine disease is underscored by recent research examining the level of disability experienced by people with migraine.[2] The study revealed that individuals with a debilitating psychological response to their condition – such as anxiety or depression – were more disabled by their migraines than those with severe and frequent attacks who maintained a positive mental outlook. It is clear that a person's psychological wellbeing can have a profound impact on their overall experience of living with migraine.

Understanding the factors that drive our brain's response to stress is essential for managing the psychological toll of migraine. By addressing these stressors, it is possible to reduce the level of disability associated with the condition and improve quality of life.

The key point to realise is that the interplay between extrinsic and intrinsic stress creates a vicious cycle. Chronic extrinsic stress can increase the frequency of migraine episodes, leading to a significant psychological toll that erodes confidence and creates intrinsic stress. This, in turn, disrupts key areas of life – such as work, family and social relationships – further intensifying extrinsic stress as these areas become harder to manage. Breaking this cycle requires a comprehensive understanding of both types of stress and their impact on the mind and body.

Figure 11 depicts how this process can contribute to the downward spiral. Extrinsic stress leads to intrinsic stress, contributing to more disability and consequently more stress. Stress can be a potent trigger for sensitisation which, of course, increases the risk of a migraine attack. Take some time to consider the three potential sources of stress and circle the ones you think may be contributing to your life's stress load.

Figure 11. The Stress Cycle

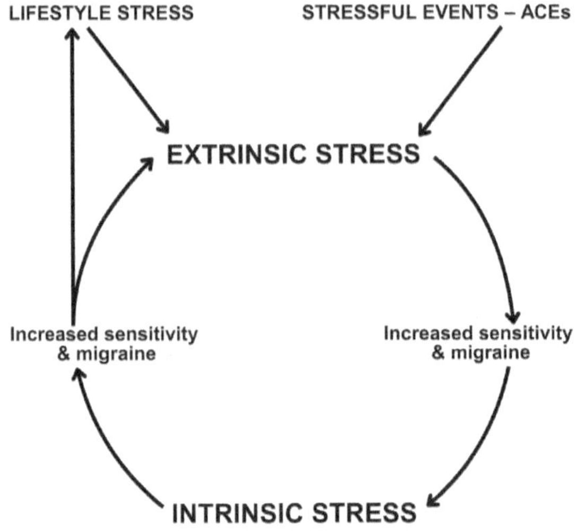

The interplay between intrinsic and extrinsic stress creates a vicious cycle.

Stress and the Migraine Brain

Understanding the complexities of how our brain functions can be a daunting task, especially without a background in psychology or neuroscience. Over the years, I've been fortunate to have many insightful conversations with Leonie Hull, co-founder of the Academy of Brain-Based Leadership. Her business partner, Dr Dan Radecki, is a neuroscientist who contributed to the development of protocols for using Botox in migraine management. Together, they use cutting-edge neuroscientific research to help create workplaces that are both productive and psychologically safe, fostering personal and collective 'psychological safety'.[3] Through my discussions with Hull – who also happens to be my sister-in-law – I've come to understand how the concept of psychological safety extends far beyond the workplace.

It's a universal principle that impacts every aspect of our lives, particularly our mental and physical health, when that sense of safety is compromised.

The Importance of Feeling Safe

I asked Hull to distil the essence of why feeling safe is so critical to our wellbeing, especially for those navigating the challenges of migraine. Her response sheds light on the profound connection between safety and our brain's survival mechanisms.

> *Over the past two million years, our brains have evolved to enhance our chances of survival – it does this by seeking safety above all else. We are literally wired for safety. The brain has learned over many trials and experiences, through many generations, how to keep us safe. These 'safety protocols' have become hardwired into our brain and the majority of the time these safety decisions happen below the level of consciousness – at a nonconscious level. This means we go into protection mode the moment our brain perceives a threat, without us even having to think about it.*
>
> *Much of this influence is controlled by the amygdala, a small but effective part of the lower or primal brain, which has the responsibility for processing emotion and responding to fear or threat.*

As you may recall from Chapter 2, the amygdala is also one of the brain regions involved in the generation of migraine. Its efficiency and potency make it a critical component of how we respond to perceived threats. In fact, it's such an effective and powerful system that politicians, marketers and the media routinely use fear to influence our thoughts and behaviour. Hull continues:

One could argue that in this day and age, we don't really need such a sensitive threat response system. This system evolved over time to keep us safe in more primitive environments where threats were predominantly physical. However, in modern society the brain has adapted this system to detect and respond to far less 'life-threatening' events like social rejection, looming deadlines or email overwhelm. These threats, while usually not a survival issue, create significant psychological discomfort.

Importantly, whilst these psychological safety threats may seem innocuous in the grand scheme of things, they can have a significant impact on our wellbeing. In fact, a 'hit' to our psychological safety can trigger a stress response that takes our higher executive brain (prefrontal cortex) offline and kicks in the SNS response. When in this triggered state, our cognition pathways are impacted, making it difficult to think, make decisions, be creative, regulate our emotions, mitigate our negativity bias and collaborate. Not to mention the negative impact it has on our mental and physical health.

The Migraine Connection

For those living with migraine, the constant intrinsic 'threat' of an attack can create a persistent sense of 'feeling unsafe'. This response often operates at a nonconscious level, such as being hyper-focused on avoiding potential triggers or scanning for early signs of an impending migraine. Even without conscious awareness, this vigilance can activate the SNS, perpetuating a cycle of stress and heightened sensitivity.

Neuroscience research has identified fundamental needs that our brain requires to feel psychologically safe. These universal needs drive our thoughts, motivations and behaviours. The Academy of Brain-Based Leadership has developed the S.A.F.E.T.Y.™ model to unpack these needs, which include Security, Autonomy, Fairness, Esteem, Trust and You. Hull elaborates on how these needs apply to individuals living with migraine and how understanding them can help foster a greater sense of safety and wellbeing:

Security

Security is our brain's need for certainty, consistency, commitment and 'no' change. Our brain is like a big prediction machine; it wants things to be 'as expected' with few surprises. It avoids the unfamiliar, dislikes change and is cautious when encountering novel situations. Any challenge to our 'security needs' is a threat to the brain and can have an incredible impact on our perceived safety.

In the migraine context, your brain's security need is constantly under threat, having very little certainty about when an attack might happen, no reliability or consistency in your environment, and the toxic undercurrent of unpredictability and change. A psychological safety landmine.

Autonomy

Autonomy is our brain's need for 'perceived' control over our lives and to have choices in things that impact us. Studies show that lack of control over your environment can dictate things like 'how much pain you feel' and 'how stress impacts you'. It also has a strong link to depression. In addition, one study showed that the biggest risk factor for high blood pressure was having a sense of helplessness, due to a perceived lack of control in our lives.

Hence, autonomy is another psychological safety need that is sabotaged for you as a migraine sufferer. You have very little control or choice in how and when an episode will hit and ultimately limited perceived control or choice in your broader life context.

Fairness

Fairness is your brain's need to experience fair exchanges, both to yourself and others. Research shows that unfairness elicits the same brain response as the powerful emotion of disgust – an important survival response to protect us from consuming poisonous substances. So, fairness is clearly of significance to our safety.

It goes without saying that if you are experiencing chronic migraine, you can have a great sense of injustice and unfairness at the suffering you, and those close to you, are enduring. This can be further exacerbated if you are going to great lengths to be proactive, seeking and following all the right advice and treatment to manage the symptoms with little or no improvement.

Esteem

Esteem is our brain's need to be highly regarded. It is derived by 'how we see ourselves', 'how we think others see us' and 'how we compare ourselves to others'. Studies show that children who suffer with low self-esteem tend to suffer with more anxiety and depression in adulthood.

Struggling with migraine can heavily impact your self-esteem, as the debilitation of the condition can mean you are frequently unable to meet work, social or relationship expectations. You can't perform at your best and are sensitive to the potential judgement and disappointment of others – which has far more impact to your brain safety than anger!

Trust

Trust is our brain's need to belong to our 'in-group'. We are social animals who thrive in social groups and communities. Our brain is wired with a strong in-group/out-group bias and is very sensitive to exclusion and rejection. In fact, research shows that the brain treats social pain the same way as it treats physical pain. However, where physical pain is difficult to recall over time, social pain can elicit the same strength of emotion experienced at the time of the event, when the memory of that event is recalled decades later.

Migraine disease can impact your ability to participate, engage and interact, leaving you feeling disconnected and excluded – relegated to the 'out-group'. This perception of 'out-group' status and the feeling of not belonging is a massive red flag to your safety.

You

Finally, the 'You' in the model is sort of the wild card. It addresses the experiences and aspects of you that make you unique. For example, your genetics, experiences, background, values, world views, current situation and plans. These factors can influence how strongly your brain responds to each of the other five S.A.F.E.T.Y.™ domains.

Understanding what these brain needs are and the potential impact they may have on you as a migraine sufferer can be helpful in demystifying some of the things you might be experiencing. It also provides a more compassionate lens to view yourself and give you keys to better identify and manage your brain's needs that are impacting you, to more effectively nurture your psychological safety.

How Does Migraine Make Us Feel 'Unsafe'?

Building on Hull's S.A.F.E.T.Y.™ framework, let's delve deeper into how the intrinsic stress of migraine develops and impacts our sense of safety.

While much attention is given to how stress can trigger migraine attacks, it's equally important to understand that living with migraine itself creates a profound psychological stress – what we refer to as intrinsic stress. This stress doesn't disappear on good days or during the interictal period (the time between migraine attacks). Even when you are not actively experiencing a migraine, the looming possibility of an attack can create a constant undercurrent of anxiety, particularly when making decisions about your future or navigating social situations.

It's not just about worrying which important life events might be disrupted by a migraine attack, it's about how this fear begins to shape your life. Many people with migraine have shared how their friends struggle to understand why they cancel plans so often. This lack of understanding can make the experience of living with migraine even more isolating and demoralising. Over time, you may find yourself avoiding social events altogether – not because you don't want to participate, but because you fear disappointing others. This withdrawal can lead to a loss of identity, as you feel increasingly defined by your condition. Research clearly shows that social disconnection exacerbates both physical pain and emotional stress.[4]

Intrinsic stress becomes so insidious, often operating below the surface without conscious awareness. In terms of psychological safety, it places you in a constant state of feeling unsafe – not just unsafe in the moment, but unsafe in planning and living your life. This is the point where your migraine disability may begin to define you. Recognising and becoming aware of this process is a crucial step in your healing journey.

This sense of vulnerability can spiral into a cycle of stress and self-doubt. Questions like, 'What if I have a migraine on the day of a family wedding or my sporting grand final?' become a persistent source of anxiety. This ongoing stress fuels the overactivation of the SNS, further eroding your confidence in your ability to 'do life'. It can affect your work or studies, causing you to fall behind, which adds external stress to the already overwhelming internal stress. The cycle deepens with every decision you face: 'Should I attend this event?' 'Should I apply for that promotion?' Over time, the frequency of these questions seems to grow alongside the frequency of your migraine episodes, creating a vicious cycle of heightened stress and more frequent attacks.

At this point, the knowledge and tools needed to regain a sense of safety can feel out of reach.

How Does Stress Trigger a Migraine Attack?

Now that we've explored how migraine creates intrinsic stress, let's examine how stress itself can trigger a migraine attack.

The amygdala, a key player in the brain's stress-response system, reacts to situations where it perceives a lack of safety. Whether it's a chronically stressful work environment or an acutely stressful event, the amygdala responds the same way – by activating the SNS response.

As part of the limbic system, the amygdala processes emotions, memories and behaviours, linking life stressors to the ANS and the HPA axis. Connections between the brainstem, limbic system and cortex, shown in Figure 12a, means that any increase in sensitivity in nerves in the brainstem and limbic system can then spread throughout the brain.

When the amygdala perceives stress as a danger, it triggers a response that ramps up the SNS. This is a normal and necessary survival mechanism designed to help us respond to threats. However, for people with migraine, this system is often overactive – see Figure 12b – creating a near-constant state of feeling 'unsafe'. This chronic activation of the SNS increases sensitivity in the brainstem and surrounding regions, potentially triggering a migraine attack.

Figure 12a. Brain Connections

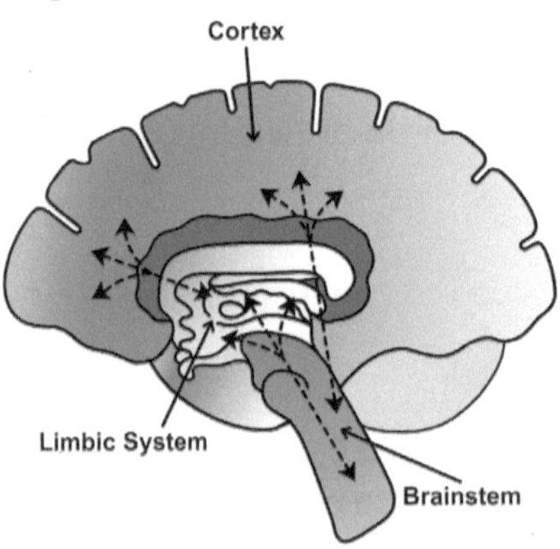

Figure 12b. Chronic Stress and Sensitisation

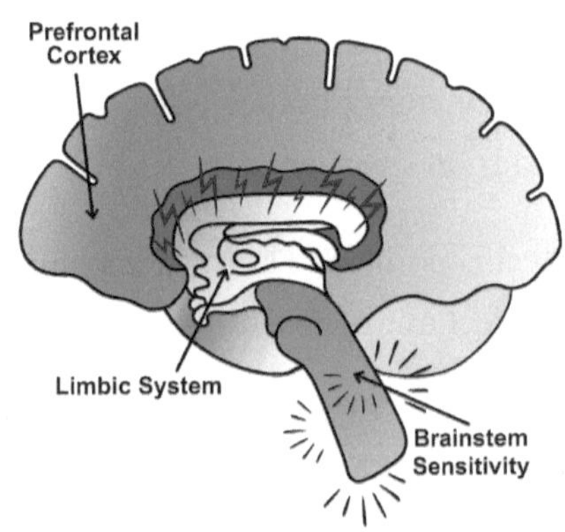

You might wonder: doesn't the brain have a mechanism to regulate the amygdala and prevent it from overwhelming the system with safety-threat messages? It does, and that mechanism is the prefrontal cortex (PFC)

Hull and Radecki explain:

> *The amygdala definitely needs a balancing response, a hand brake if you like, so it doesn't create havoc in your brain. It's called the prefrontal cortex (PFC) and is a newer part of your brain from an evolutionary point of view. It is not as efficient as the lower nonconscious part of your brain in processing information. It takes more resources such as energy stores in the brain to do its work, so it is prone to fatiguing quicker than the amygdala which just powers on regardless.*
>
> *In the context of migraine and stress, the PFC should be working to calm down the ANS to enable you to make rational, balanced responses to perceived threats. The problem is that when the PFC begins to fade and fatigue, which it will inevitably do, the amygdala can become too influential than what is ideal.*

If the PFC sounds familiar, it's because this is the same area of the brain inhibited by cortical spreading depression (CSD), a phenomenon linked to migraine attacks. If the PFC is prone to fatigue in a typical brain, imagine how much more vulnerable it is in a migraine brain, where it may also be affected by CSD. This is why the amygdala and limbic system have such a strong influence on the generation of migraine attacks.[5-7]

The functional connections of the amygdala and brainstem, including the upper neck,[8] means that issues in one area of the brain can ripple outward, affecting the entire lower brain region. This interconnected system underscores the complexity of migraine and highlights the importance of addressing both the physical and psychological aspects of the condition.

My Stress and Its Impact on the Migraine Journey

For many who experience migraine, stress often coincides with an increase in frequency or intensity. Reflecting on my own journey, I can see how chronic stress and a traumatic event contributed to my struggles with migraine.

I've always led a busy life, a work ethic instilled in me by my parents. However, this constant busyness was never balanced with downtime or mindfulness practices. Over 15 years, this relentless pace took a toll on my nervous system. I vividly recall countless nights waking up stressed, sweating over decisions or unresolved issues – clear signs of an SNS stuck in overdrive.

Life with a young family only added to the chaos. Between school, sports and community commitments, there was never a moment to slow down. Relaxation only came during holidays, offering a brief pause. One silver lining of the COVID-19 pandemic was the collective lesson that it's okay to slow down.[9] *Yet, as life has returned to its pre-pandemic pace, this lesson seems to have faded.*

The turning point came on December 10th, 2000 – six months after my migraine episodes had started to become more frequent. It was a relaxed Sunday by the pool with friends, a hot summer day that turned into a nightmare. My three-year-old son, Hayden, was found floating face-down in the water. He was unresponsive, not breathing, his teeth clenched, and frothing at the mouth. Thankfully, I resuscitated him, and within moments he was back to his usual self. However, the trauma of those 15 minutes has stayed with me for over 25 years. Pool parties became a source of immense stress, and water safety remains deeply ingrained in my psyche.

This event pushed my ANS into sympathetic overdrive. In this state, the SNS is constantly activated, while the PNS struggles to restore balance. Living in this state of constant agitation, anxiety, fatigue and poor sleep became my new normal. This inevitably increased the frequency and intensity of my migraine attacks.

In hindsight, this traumatic event likely did more to lock me into SNS overdrive than any other factor in my life. However, my pre-existing chronic stress from a busy lifestyle certainly didn't help. From that day in December 2000, migraine became the dominant health issue in my life. With little more than anti-nausea medication and sleep as my tools for coping, I was ill-equipped to manage the condition.

Research draws attention to a significant gap in the psychological treatment of migraine: the lack of focus on addressing past traumatic events.[10] While cognitive and mindfulness-based practices can be helpful, they often fail to address the maladaptive responses people develop following major life stressors. This blind spot in my own migraine journey – daily stress compounded by a traumatic event – was a major factor in my downward spiral.

What began as an insidious build-up of stress from a busy life was ultimately pushed over the edge by one traumatic event. The result was eight years of regular, debilitating migraine attacks. But the impact wasn't limited to the attacks themselves. During this period, my overall quality of life suffered significantly, even in the times between migraine attacks.

Three Psychological Stages of the Downward Spiral

Reflecting on my experience with migraine as a disease, I've identified three distinct psychological stages that shaped my journey. With the benefit of hindsight and education, I now understand how the intrinsic and extrinsic stress cycle contributed to my downward spiral. At the time, however, I was so consumed by the experience that I couldn't see a way out. Over the past 15 years, I've observed similar patterns in many migraine patients, leading me to believe this is a common experience among migraine sufferers.

Stage 1: Living in Ignorance

When migraine first becomes a regular part of your life, the lack of understanding about what's happening can be deeply unsettling. You may find yourself wondering what has changed to make migraine such a significant issue. During the initial severe episodes, many people end up in the emergency department because the symptoms are so debilitating. After undergoing extensive tests, including brain scans, you're often reassured that there's no life-threatening condition, such as a tumour. While this reassurance is meant to provide comfort, it can sometimes have the opposite effect. Without a clear explanation of what migraine is or why they're worsening, the uncertainty can fuel anxiety.

This anxiety, in turn, can heighten the SNS response, creating a vicious cycle of stress and worsening symptoms. The lack of understanding leaves you feeling lost and powerless, unable to grasp what's happening or how to regain control.

Stage 2: Understanding but Helpless

Receiving a diagnosis of migraine can bring initial relief. Knowing what's wrong – and confirming it's not something more serious, like a brain tumour – can alleviate some of the anxiety caused by ignorance. However, this relief is often short-lived. Understanding the condition is only the first step; finding effective treatment is a much longer and more challenging process.

Starting a treatment program and experiencing some improvement can boost your psychological outlook. However, for many, the journey to effective treatment is arduous. Medications often require months of trial and error to determine their effectiveness, and even when they work, side effects can be a significant drawback. Finding the right combination of medications can be a prolonged and frustrating process.

Some people turn to identifying triggers, hoping to pinpoint what causes their migraine attacks. While this approach can be helpful, it's often slow and not always conclusive. As time passes with minimal progress, a sense of helplessness can set in. The constant focus on managing migraine can lead to hyper-vigilance, making you feel unsafe and on edge. This heightened state of awareness can activate the amygdala response, further exacerbating the psychological toll.

Stage 3: Losing Yourself to Migraine

Over time, migraine can become so overwhelming that it can dominate your life. After months, or even years, of uncertainty and experimentation, you may feel no closer to finding answers. The intrinsic stress of living with migraine can take a toll, leaving you feeling as though you've lost yourself to the 'migraine life'.

This loss of identity is both physical and psychological. Research has shown that the interictal burden of migraine – the impact it has between attacks – can significantly affect quality of life.[11] Migraine influences every aspect of life, from physical and emotional wellbeing to cognitive and social functioning. As these key areas of life are affected, it can feel as though your identity is being eroded by a disease you can't control, further damaging your psychological health.

Moving Forward with Empowerment

A recent study revealed that a higher interictal burden is often linked to dissatisfaction with treatment and depression.[11] This connection is understandable, as feeling powerless over migraine attacks and experiencing limited success with treatment can make it challenging to stay optimistic about the future. Therefore, discovering an effective treatment approach that empowers you with greater control can lead to significant psychological and physical benefits.

As the saying goes, knowledge is power. Recognising these psychological stages is the first step towards empowerment. By understanding your journey, you can begin to take control with specific approaches that make a difference. Psychological support may be particularly helpful if you feel like you're losing your identity to migraine.

Journalling can be a valuable tool for reflecting on your psychological journey. Writing down your thoughts can provide clarity about the road you've travelled and help you plan a pathway forward. As we move into the final stage of this book, remember to be kind to yourself. The journey so far has been incredibly challenging, but it's not a reflection of failure – it's simply the reality of living with chronic pain.

The Destructive Nature of Chronic Pain

Chronic pain and mental health are closely interconnected. A recent study emphasised the bi-directional relationship between chronic pain – such as headaches, neck pain and insomnia – and mental health.[12] The findings underscore the importance of addressing both physical and psychological factors when managing chronic pain. Pain catastrophising, a common issue in migraine, often amplifies pain intensity and disability.[13] In my experience, psychological interventions remain an underutilised tool in managing these aspects of migraine.

Further supporting this perspective is the observation that symptoms of anxiety and depression are more prevalent in children with migraine, indicating that these mental health patterns may develop early in life.[14] Cultivating a healthy psychological outlook from a young age, both in general and in relation to pain, could significantly influence whether an individual is defined by their migraine condition or maintains an identity independent of it.

Benefits of Psychological Treatment for Migraine

If you are experiencing the profound psychological effects of a downward spiral, take comfort in knowing there are positive steps you can take to begin your journey towards a better life. Often, the first steps involve addressing psychological factors, such as shifting your mindset to focus on positive options. This process may include recognising and understanding your subconscious responses to migraine. For instance, you might notice that you are withdrawing from social events. Once you identify this pattern, you can take proactive and mindful steps to address it.

Psychological interventions can effectively target issues such as social disconnection, anxiety and pain catastrophising.[4,13,15] Research suggests that these psychological factors are stronger predictors of the level of disability experienced by individuals with migraine than the frequency or intensity of the migraines themselves.[16] Therefore, managing these psychological variables can significantly reduce the level of disability associated with migraine disease.

In fact, substantial research demonstrates that psychological interventions can positively impact not only disability levels but also migraine frequency and intensity.[17,18] For example, one study incorporated mindfulness training alongside standard medication in a trial where half of the participants received only medication. The group that combined mindfulness with medication experienced significantly better outcomes, including reduced disability, lower headache frequency, improved quality of life and decreased anxiety levels.[19]

Future research should focus on testing combinations of two or more treatments to determine whether integrated approaches yield superior results.

Conclusion

Intrinsic stress is an issue that develops with ongoing migraine disability, which begins to create roadblocks to a person just doing normal life. Understanding the processes involved gives you the knowledge you need to start clearing the pathway so you can move forward in life.

Even if psychological interventions result in only small to moderate improvements in managing migraine, they represent meaningful progress. When these gains are combined with other interventions that also yield small to moderate benefits, the cumulative effect can create significant momentum towards better health outcomes.

This approach aligns with the biopsychosocial model of treatment, widely regarded as the gold standard in the health sector. This model takes a holistic view of health, addressing the physical, psychological and social aspects of a person's wellbeing.

In the next section of the book, we will explore how this model can be applied to your unique situation as someone affected by migraine. We will delve into holistic treatment options that address various lifestyle factors potentially influencing your migraine experience. The ultimate aim is to reduce brainstem sensitivity and help you build a strong support team to guide you towards a healthier, more fulfilling life.

It's time to take the first steps on your pathway to improvement.

03

Chapter 7:

Pathways to Improvement – The Holistic Approach

Chapter 8:

Start Walking – The Road to Better Health

Chapter 9:

Embracing Change – Moving Towards a Better Future

SECTION 3

The Plan

CHAPTER 7

Pathways to Improvement

The Holistic Approach

We've all experienced moments in medical care where we feel reduced to just an injury or illness, rather than being recognised as a whole person. Our unique needs, aspirations and the life we've built – centred around family, friends, work and future goals – can often feel invisible in these situations. This approach can feel absurd. For instance, individuals with knee pain on stairs have shared that their medical advice was simply to avoid stairs altogether. Similarly, for those living with migraine, the advice to avoid potential triggers – like exercise or work-related travel – can feel equally impractical, especially when these activities are essential to maintaining a fulfilling and balanced life.

Unfortunately, this fragmented approach has become a norm in modern medicine, where every issue is divided up into specialties. This system, although beneficial for improved quality of care for a specific health issue, can lead to depersonalisation and inefficiency. If not balanced with a more complete view of a person's health needs, it ultimately affects the quality of care being offered.

The future of healthcare should ideally embrace a holistic approach as the benchmark for all medical services. This approach empowers individuals with knowledge, enabling them to make positive changes in their lives. A medical model that prioritises holistic health naturally fosters happiness and a sense of safety.

The holistic approach has been gaining momentum in the medical community over the past 50 years. Known as the biopsychosocial (BPS) model, it has been part of the World Health Organization's (WHO) definition of health since 1948.[1] The BPS model considers a person's biology, psychology, social and environmental circumstances when addressing medical issues. It shifts the focus from merely treating a condition to improving the overall health and wellbeing of the individual.

In this chapter, we aim to determine your starting point on this holistic health journey through a five-step evaluation plan – not just focusing on your migraine but on your overall health. Remember we want to avoid hypervigilance and the stress it may evoke as it may lead to heightened stress and a worsening of your migraine presentation. It's essential to avoid letting migraine define you. A holistic approach centred on your health as well as your migraine presentation can help you achieve this balance.

This proactive model of care is designed to help the whole person thrive – biologically, psychologically and socially – rather than merely survive from one medical episode to the next. My hope is that this book will guide you towards this approach, empowering you to take control of your health with the support of family, friends and a dedicated medical team. Together, you can overcome the limitations that migraine imposes and begin to truly thrive.

As you approach your five-step evaluation plan, here are some key points to help you stay focused and avoid feeling overwhelmed:

- Migraine is a complex neurological disorder, but it doesn't have to feel daunting. It simply means your genetics amplify the brain's response to normal sensory input, making the nerves more reactive.
- Migraine is not a one-size-fits-all condition. Every person's experience is unique, and it's important to be comfortable with the uncertainty of how your migraine will respond to the interventions outlined in this chapter.
- While your genetic makeup is the underlying cause of migraine, lifestyle and environmental factors can exacerbate the condition. You now understand the importance of addressing these factors alongside exploring treatment options beyond medication, with the support of an experienced healthcare team.

Rethinking Migraine Treatment

Historically, migraine treatment has relied heavily on the biomedical model, which centres on biological factors and often prioritises medication as the primary solution.[1] While medications can be effective, the notion that a single tablet or injection can resolve all migraine-related issues is misleading. This phenomenon, where a patient experiences exceptional results, is known as the 'super responder' effect, but it is far from the norm.

A super responder is defined as someone with migraine who experiences a greater than 75% reduction in monthly headache days (MHD) by the third month after starting a new medication or treatment. A recent study on a newer CGRP (calcitonin gene-related peptide) medication revealed that 11% of participants were super responders, while 10% were non-responders, achieving less than a 25% reduction in MHD.[2] These statistics show that 80% of individuals fall somewhere between these two extremes.

While CGRP medications have been revolutionary for some, it is clear they are not the ultimate solution for everyone.

In fact, a migraine medication is considered effective if it reduces headache days by 50% for half of its users. This benchmark is lower than the standard for many medications, reflecting the complex and multifactorial nature of migraine. As discussed throughout this book, migraine disease is influenced by a combination of genetic, environmental and lifestyle factors, making it challenging to treat, especially with a one-size-fits-all approach.

So, why is the focus on medications? There are two primary reasons why migraine treatment has been predominantly medication-driven:

- **The genetic perspective**: Migraine is often classified as a genetic condition, leading to the belief that it cannot be cured and must be managed with medication. Like many other health conditions, lifestyle and environmental factors in migraine need to be addressed alongside medications for optimal outcomes.
- **Research limitations:** Conducting effective research on a complex condition like migraine requires large participant numbers, which is more feasible and cost-effective with medication trials. Comparing a drug to a placebo, such as a sugar pill, is straightforward compared to assessing diet, neck treatment or psychological factors.

The Biopsychosocial (BPS) Model

Using a one-pronged approach to address a multifactorial problem seems illogical. This is why the BPS model is a more effective approach. It encourages a multi-component treatment plan involving a multidisciplinary team of trained health professionals. Unlike social media influencers promoting unproven remedies, these professionals assess and address individual needs, recognising the complexity of migraine management.

Categorising treatment pathways into biological, psychological and social domains can be challenging, as many factors overlap. For example, sleep impacts both physical and psychological health but is also influenced by stress and social circumstances. Similarly, diet is a lifestyle choice affected by mental outlook, physical health and social environment.

As discussed in Chapter 4, the genetics–lifestyle–environmental cake analogy illustrates how these components interact. Just as the ingredients, recipe and cooking conditions combine to create a cake, the interplay of genetic, lifestyle and environmental factors determines migraine outcomes. Once a cake is baked, the components cannot be separated, but the recipe can be adjusted for better results next time.

And it's the same with migraine. When your brainstem becomes sensitised beyond a certain threshold, it triggers a migraine. Tweaking one component may have a small effect on the final result, such as reducing migraine frequency. However, tweaking multiple components in tandem will have a dramatic effect on the final result. The bonus is, in most cases, even if tweaking one of these components doesn't change your migraine presentation it will likely still improve your health.

The key is that just as every migraine presentation is different, the holistic intervention program for each individual needs to be different, tailored to that person's particular biopsychosocial needs.[3] Just because someone says they responded well to a particular intervention doesn't mean you will too. This is why you need to be structured and systematic in the way you integrate the BPS interventions into your life.

A Five-Step Framework

To make this process more structured and manageable, we'll establish a framework with five steps to guide you, so it won't feel like 'mission impossible'. These steps will help you choose interventions that are more likely to yield positive results. This initial phase is crucial because seeing prompt, positive changes can provide the motivation needed to continue on this journey. Journalling the process can be invaluable, allowing you to revisit and refine your approach as new insights emerge.

Here's a summary of the five steps that will get you started:

Step 1: Review Your Current Situation and Identify Key Issues

Step 2: Map Your Journey on the Stress Cycle Graph

Step 3: Choose a Measurable Health or Migraine Issue

Step 4: Identify Your Triggers

Step 5: Plan and Prioritise Interventions

Hopefully, you have been carefully considering areas of change as you have been progressing through this book. By doing so, you'll be better equipped to take control of your migraine disease and health. Remember, this is a journey, and every small step forward is progress.

Where We Can Intervene

This five-step plan will address the following pathways to improvement. Remind yourself of these potential pathways and highlight two or three that you think are most likely to be of benefit to you.

- **Genetics/epigenetics:** While we can't change our genetics, we can influence our epigenetics. Lifestyle and environmental factors play a significant role in how genes are expressed, impacting your migraine presentation.
- **Look back to your youth:** Reflecting on childhood health issues can reveal underlying factors contributing to migraine presentation. It may also uncover unresolved health challenges you haven't addressed, such as psychological responses to trauma.
- **Environment:** Your living environment can influence migraine. While relocating may not always be feasible, understanding environmental triggers can help you make informed decisions.
- **Lifestyle:** Diet and stress management are critical. These factors significantly impact the gut-brain axis, which can either heighten or reduce brainstem sensitivity, depending on the quality of your diet and the suitability of your response to stress.
- **Activity/exercise:** Regular activity and exercise can improve mental outlook, reduce stress, enhance sleep quality and lower the risk of vascular diseases, all of which can positively influence your migraine presentation and general health.
- **Symptom triggers:** Identifying and managing triggers such as specific foods, weather changes, smells or poor sleep requires a systematic and dedicated approach.
- **Hormones:** Hormonal fluctuations are a significant factor, particularly for women, who experience migraine at a rate three times higher than men. Addressing hormonal influences can be challenging but also essential where this is a major contributing factor.

- **Medication overuse:** Overusing acute headache medications, such as over-the-counter analgesics or triptans, can lead to chronic migraine. It may also contribute to gut issues and increased central sensitisation.
- **Upper neck:** The upper neck, specifically the top three vertebral levels (C1–C3) and the occipital triangle muscles, has a direct impact on brainstem sensitivity. Past injuries, such as whiplash or concussion, can cause long-term dysfunction, aggravating migraine.
- **The stress of migraine:** The intrinsic stress associated with migraine can create a vicious cycle, amplifying pain and frequency. Addressing all aspects of psychological stress is a vital component of the holistic approach.

The Five Steps to Start Your Journey

Taking the first steps to manage migraine disease can feel daunting, especially if you're in survival mode. However, planning your journey to better health is an essential step towards regaining control. Think of this as a stocktake of your current health and migraine situation. While it may seem overwhelming, this process will help you identify the best pathway to begin your journey.

Even if you already have a clear idea of where to start, it's still worth completing this five-step review. It will not only solidify your initial plan but also prepare you for potential second and third interventions down the line.

Step 1: Review Your Current Situation and Identify Key Issues

Start by summarising the frequency, intensity and duration of your migraine episodes, along with any associated symptoms. If you haven't been keeping a migraine diary, now is the time to start. While documenting your episodes may feel like the last thing you want to do, it's essential for tracking patterns and evaluating the effectiveness of interventions. Without this information, it's easy to overlook subtle changes or misjudge the severity of your condition.

Reflect on the past few years and consider factors such as medication changes, childhood illnesses and family medical history. What treatments or strategies have you tried in the past? Were they beneficial? Documenting this information will help you build a comprehensive history of your migraine disease, which will be invaluable as you move forward.

Once you've reviewed your history, create a short list of possible key issues that you believe need to be addressed. These could be based on your research, intuition or discussions with your healthcare provider. Here is a list of potential issues you may need to address:

- **Environmental factors**
  - Where do you live?
  - How is your sleep quality?
  - What stress is impacting your life?
- **Lifestyle factors**
  - Dietary aspects
  - Stress response (extrinsic and intrinsic)
  - Exercise
  - Hormonal influence

* Medication overuse
* Upper neck dysfunction
* Triggers

Step 2: Map Your Journey on the Stress Cycle Graph

Stress is a significant factor in migraine management. To understand its impact, consider three key areas:

1. Major stressful events

2. Daily lifestyle stress

3. Intrinsic stress caused by migraine

If stress is a major issue for you, seeking psychological support could be a critical pathway. Studies have shown that individuals with a positive psychological outlook experience less migraine-related disability and cope more effectively with episodes.[4]

Be specific about which aspects of stress are most significant for you. If you're already receiving psychological support, note whether there are areas that remain unaddressed. Refer back to Chapter 6 where you may have already highlighted which three key areas could be involved in your life stress. Take a moment now to map out your stress on the Stress Cycle graph in Figure 13, so you can visualise patterns and identify areas for intervention.

Figure 13. The Stress Cycle

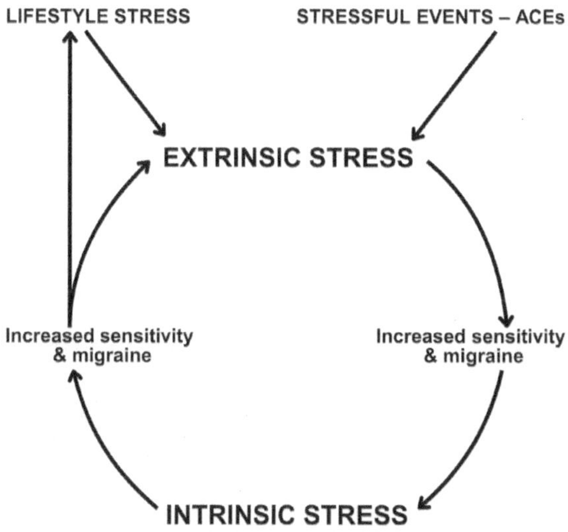

Step 3: Choose a Measurable Health or Migraine Issue

Do you have a health problem, family history or comorbidity associated with migraine? Conditions such as cardiovascular disease, EDS/hypermobility, behavioural disorders (e.g. ADD/ADHD), allergic reactions, ANS dysfunction or sleep disruption can all be linked to migraine.[5] Identifying these connections can help you prioritise interventions that address both migraine and related health issues.

For example, if poor sleep is a major driver of your migraine attacks, understanding the root cause of your sleep disruption would be a logical starting point. Similarly, if you have cardiovascular concerns, incorporating exercise into your routine could benefit both your general health and migraine presentation.

Track objective health measures, such as blood test results (e.g. cholesterol or glucose levels) or wellness questionnaires. These metrics, combined with your migraine diary, can help you monitor progress and stay motivated.

Step 4: Identify Your Triggers

Create a list of potential migraine triggers, even if you're not entirely certain they cause your attacks. Triggers often work in combination, making it difficult to pinpoint exact causes. However, identifying patterns can help you prioritise interventions. If you feel this is an area you'd like to explore further, make a note of it. Understanding your triggers can be a key step in reducing the frequency and severity of your migraine episodes.

Step 5: Plan and Prioritise Interventions

Using the insights from the previous steps, create a list of possible interventions and prioritise them. Always consult with your doctor to review your health and medical concerns, as they can provide valuable insights and recommend additional tests if needed.

Choose an intervention that feels manageable and directly addresses your migraine presentation or a related health issue. If you have multiple options, prioritise one that may also benefit a comorbidity. Start small to avoid feeling overwhelmed. For example, if exercise is your chosen intervention, begin with three 15-minute walks per week for four weeks. Once you've established a routine, you can gradually build on it.

The Italian concept of 'make haste slowly' is particularly relevant here. Set small, achievable goals that fit into your lifestyle, especially if you're low on energy or time. Be kind to yourself and focus on steady, sustainable progress.

By following these five steps, you'll create a clear and actionable plan to manage your migraine disease and improve your overall health. Remember, every small step forward is a step towards better wellbeing.

My Discovery of New Pathways for Migraine Treatment

The evolution of a more holistic approach to migraine treatment has been a gradual yet transformative journey for me as a practitioner. Over time, our headache centres have been steadily transitioning towards a biopsychosocial model of care. This shift was accelerated by our exploration into concussion management and, unexpectedly, by a brief but impactful trip to England.

It was late May 2019, and I was meeting my sisters in our old hometown of High Wycombe, Buckinghamshire, England. Mum, Dad and my sisters had lived in this town for eight years. My brother and I were born there, and we were heading back to spread Mum's ashes with some old friends who were unable to make it out to her funeral.

While in the UK, I visited Australian friends Mick and Briony[4]*, who had been living in London for nearly a decade. Mick had developed a strong interest in optimising his health and shared his experiences with interventions like intermittent fasting, cold therapy (even cold showers in the harsh London winter), slow deep breathing exercises to manage stress, and heart rate-focused exercise. These strategies were aimed at calming the autonomic nervous system (ANS) and reducing brain inflammation. This*

4 Mick and Briony are good friends (names changed for privacy) who have kindly given their consent to be reference in this book.

resonated deeply with me as these interventions aligned with the CCMI approach to concussion rehabilitation that I had become interested in. I began to contemplate if this could be relevant to migraine treatment as well.

Inspired by these discussions, I made immediate changes upon returning to Sydney. I began winter swims at Cronulla Beach, something I had previously avoided due to concerns about falling ill. I also experimented with intermittent fasting and relaxation techniques, particularly slow breathing exercises, to observe their effects on my 'migraine brain'.

After my return from the UK, I delved deeper into the parallels between concussion and migraine. I was struck by the shared challenges: ANS dysregulation, inflammation, visual and vestibular disturbances, balance issues, neck dysfunction and psychological disruption. Research confirmed the presence of these issues in migraine patients, and I was encouraged to find that many alternative brain health interventions had already been trialled for migraine. Evidence supported the benefits of exercise, dietary changes and relaxation or mindfulness techniques for managing migraine disease.

A Practical Example: Sarah's Journey to Managing Migraine

Now that you've seen the five steps, let's take a closer look at how they might play out, using a fictional example of a woman called Sarah.

Step 1: Review Current Situation and Identify Key Issues

When Sarah, a 35-year-old professional, reviews her history, she identifies several key details:

- *She experiences migraine twice a month, with an intensity of 7–9/10 lasting 6–8 hours.*
- *Her family history includes migraine among her sister, mother and aunts, as well as strokes in her grandmother and great-grandmother.*
- *Sarah recalls a significant abdominal illness during childhood, which may have coincided with the onset of her migraine attacks.*
- *Initially, over-the-counter medications like Nurofen and Panadol were effective, but they no longer provide relief. Her migraine symptoms now include nausea, vomiting and light sensitivity, forcing her to retreat to a dark, quiet room for hours.*
- *Migraine often occurs at the start of her menstrual cycle, though not exclusively.*
- *Her stressful job, particularly during deadlines, disrupts her sleep, leaving her tired and affecting her productivity.*
- *Despite her positive outlook, Sarah is increasingly frustrated by the growing intensity and frequency of her migraine attacks.*

Sarah's list of possible issues to address:

- *Minimise stroke risk factors due to her genetic history.*
- *Investigate potential gut issues linked to her childhood illness.*
- *Manage chronic and intrinsic stress.*
- *Explore hormonal factors.*
- *Consider medication overuse headache as a contributing factor.*

Step 2: Map Your Journey on the Stress Cycle Graph

Using the Stress Cycle Graph shown in Figure 14, Sarah identifies that while her work deadlines contribute to extrinsic stress, she is not yet experiencing significant intrinsic stress. However, her growing frustration with migraine suggests she is nearing that point. Her positive attitude has likely helped mitigate intrinsic stress so far.

Figure 14. Sarah's Stress Cycle Graph

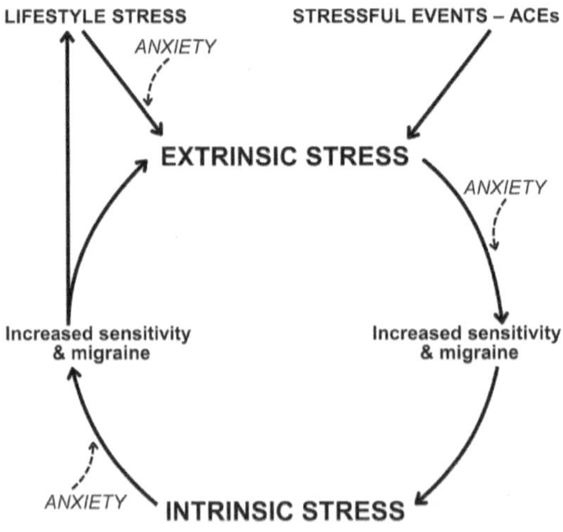

Sarah's list of potential stress interventions:

- *Implement simple stress-management techniques during work deadlines.*
- *Focus on strategies that also improve sleep quality, particularly during high-stress periods.*

Step 3: Choose a Measurable Health or Migraine Issue

Sarah's review highlights two potential comorbidities:

- *Family history of stroke*
- *Abdominal issues, possibly linked to gut intolerances or allergies*

After consulting her doctor, Sarah prioritises addressing her family history of stroke. Together, she and her doctor identify key measurements to monitor:

- *Blood pressure*
- *Blood glucose*
- *Cholesterol levels*
- *BMI*

Sarah decides to focus on regular blood tests and monitoring her BMI, as she has noticed weight gain due to stress and poor dietary habits.

Step 4: Identify Your Triggers

Sarah identifies several potential migraine triggers:

- *Hormonal changes, particularly at the start of her menstrual cycle*

- *Diet, including rich foods and junk food*
- *Bright lights, such as driving at night*

While these triggers are not always consistent, they provide a starting point for intervention.

Step 5: Plan and Prioritise Interventions

Sarah decides to start with simpler interventions to avoid feeling overwhelmed, especially given her demanding job.

Priority 1 ***Address Daily Stress***

Action *Consult a psychologist and learn meditation techniques. This feels like a manageable first step and is less likely to add to her stress.*

Priority 2 ***Improve Sleep Quality***

Action *Build on her meditation practice to relax before bed and explore other sleep-improvement strategies. If these changes are insufficient, Sarah's doctor has suggested a sleep study as a next step.*

Priority 3 ***Focus on Dietary Issues***

Action *Gradually reduce junk food intake and investigate potential food intolerances or allergies. This may also help address her stroke risk and childhood gut issues.*

Priority 4 ***Investigate Hormonal Contributions***

Action *While Sarah suspects hormones play a role, she is hesitant to track and journal. She decides to explore this area only if other strategies prove ineffective.*

By taking a structured, step-by-step approach, Sarah can address her migraine disease in a way that feels manageable and sustainable. The Migraine Threshold Graph in Figure 15 demonstrates how small changes in a number of areas can reduce her sensitivity, even without addressing hormonal issues. Assuming her interventions each have some small positive effect, she will effectively raise her migraine threshold and reduce the risk of a migraine attack. This process allows her to focus on the most pressing issues first while leaving room to explore other factors as needed.

Figure 15. Migraine Threshold: Sarah's Goal

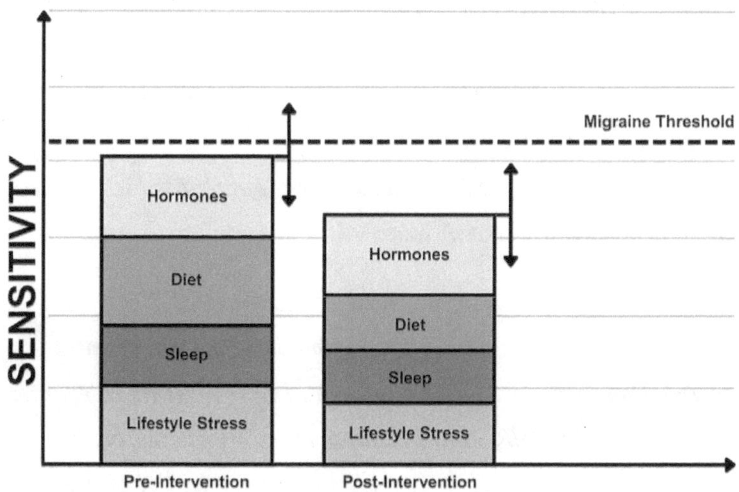

The impact of a multifaceted approach to migraine treatment for Sarah.

My Initial Intervention

The first treatment I explored was addressing my neck, as it appeared to play a role in the onset of migraine. At the time, this seemed like a logical starting point, although I was unaware of the many other options available to manage migraine disability. Triptan-based medications, introduced in the 1990s, were still not widely understood by the early 2000s, except by a small number of headache specialists.

In my case, neck treatment appeared to have a significant impact. Over time, I noticed a reduction in the frequency and severity of my migraine episodes. While I continued to experience morning headaches at the back of my head, they no longer progressed to full-blown migraine attacks. Keeping a headache diary could have made this improvement evident sooner, but the changes eventually became clear.

This initial intervention provided a much-needed break from regular migraine episodes, allowing me to regain energy and motivation to explore additional steps. Improvements in my diet and exercise, initially aimed at supporting my overall health, also appeared to contribute to reducing the sensitivity of my migraine brain. Over the years, with multiple interventions, I have experienced fewer migraine episodes, with a noticeable reduction in their intensity and associated symptoms.

NOTE: Remember that your experience will, most likely, be very different to mine. Don't set your expectations too high from the start. The research for all possible interventions is credible but still needs to be applied to you, in your unique situation.

Your Holistic Approach to Migraine Management

A migraine occurs when the brainstem becomes sensitised to a certain threshold. Adjusting one factor, such as diet or stress, may yield modest improvements. However, addressing multiple factors can lead to significant changes in migraine frequency and severity. Even if an adjustment to one factor does not directly impact your migraine presentation, it is likely to improve your overall health.

The key is recognising that every migraine presentation is unique, requiring a tailored intervention program that addresses your specific biopsychosocial needs.[3] By moving away from a one-pronged, medication-focused approach and embracing a holistic model, you can find a more effective and sustainable approach to living with migraine.

The Ultimate Goal is Desensitisation

The primary aim of any migraine intervention is to reduce the sensitivity of the brainstem region, which plays a central role in regulating essential bodily functions and processing sensory input. When the brainstem becomes overly reactive, it can trigger a cascade of neurological events that lead to a migraine attack. Therefore, the ultimate goal is to make the migraine brain more resilient to the various triggers and stressors – such as environmental changes, hormonal fluctuations or lifestyle factors – that can push it into 'migraine mode', initiating an attack.

Achieving this resilience requires the brain to undergo a process of rewiring, which involves modifying the neurological pathways associated with migraine. This rewiring helps to block or dampen the overactive signals that contribute to the onset of an attack. However, the extent to which this can be achieved depends on individual factors, including your genetic makeup, overall health and unique circumstances. No two migraine experiences are the same, and as such, interventions must be tailored to address the specific needs of each individual.

This transformation is not an overnight process; it demands a systematic, patient and persistent approach. The brain is essentially 'unlearning' an ingrained habit of heightened sensitivity while simultaneously learning a new skill – how to remain calm and less reactive to potential triggers. This requires consistent effort, whether through lifestyle adjustments, dietary changes, stress management techniques or medical interventions. It's important to remember that progress may be gradual, and setbacks are a natural part of the journey. However, with time, dedication and the right support, it is possible to build a more resilient brain and reduce the frequency and severity of migraine episodes.

Moving Towards a Multifaceted Treatment Plan

Adopting a holistic treatment approach for migraine may require some mental adjustments. While the approach is multifaceted, it's important to focus on one factor at a time, making progress in that area before introducing another. This gradual process is designed to fine-tune enough factors to reduce brainstem sensitisation, ultimately lowering the likelihood of reaching your migraine threshold, as shown in Figure 16.

Figure 16. Migraine Threshold: a Practical Example

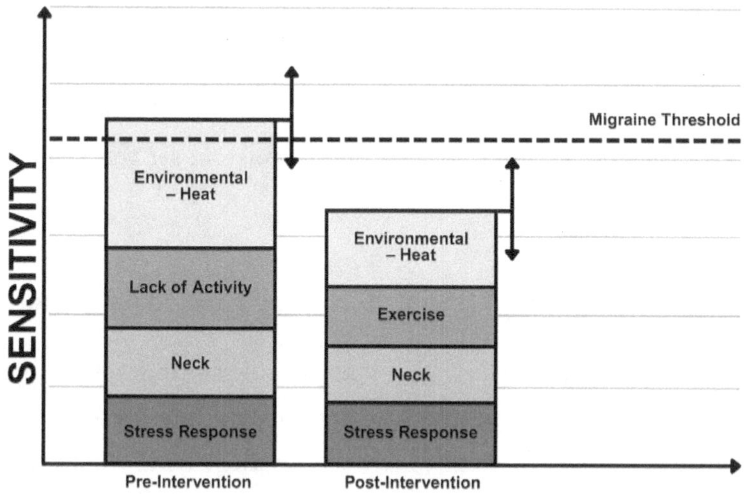

The impact of a multifaceted approach to migraine treatment achieving small improvements in several areas.

These factors can influence various aspects of sensitisation, such as neuro-inflammation, epigenetics, vascular health, or reducing painful stimuli. Over time, the cumulative effect of these small, positive changes can create a significant impact on your migraine experience – a phenomenon known as the 'multiplier effect'.

It's crucial to remember that if the first factor you address doesn't yield a major improvement, it may still play a vital role in the bigger picture. Each step contributes to the overall goal of reducing brainstem sensitivity and building resilience against migraine triggers. Patience and persistence are key as you work towards a more manageable and balanced life with migraine.

Common Pitfalls to Avoid

Starting a new approach to managing your migraine condition can be both exciting and daunting. However, there are two common pitfalls that can hinder your progress and dampen your motivation early on. By understanding and addressing these points, you can set yourself up for a smoother and more successful journey.

Track Your Headaches Without Becoming Fixated on Them

Keeping a headache diary is an essential tool for understanding your migraine patterns. Migraine attacks often vary in their presentation, and tracking these changes over time is crucial for identifying what works and what doesn't. Without this information, it can be difficult to gauge your progress or pinpoint effective strategies.

There are several migraine apps, such as Migraine Buddy and Migraine Monitor, that can help you log your episodes, potential triggers and medication effects. These apps are designed to simplify the process and prevent you from overanalysing every detail of your headache days. While it's important to record significant changes in your symptoms, avoid obsessing over every moment of discomfort. Over-focusing on your pain can inadvertently amplify it.

Remember, even small changes in your migraine patterns can signal progress. Use your diary as a tool for insight, not as a source of stress.

Ease into Change To Avoid Flare-Ups

The migraine brain is highly sensitive and reactive, often perceiving change as a threat. This heightened state, driven by the amygdala, can trigger a migraine attack in response to sudden or drastic changes. To avoid this, it's essential to introduce new habits gradually.

For instance, if you're planning to improve your diet, start small. Focus on modifying one meal at a time or eliminating a single food group. Abrupt changes, such as starting a ketogenic diet and cutting out all carbohydrates overnight, can overwhelm your system and provoke a migraine response.

Similarly, if you're incorporating exercise into your routine, begin at your current fitness level and build up slowly. Your brain needs time to adapt to new routines, and a gentle approach will help minimise the risk of triggering an attack.

Above all, be kind to yourself – managing migraine is a journey, not a race. Progress may be slow, but with patience and persistence, your brain pathways will adapt to the changes you introduce.

Conclusion

As you embark on this journey to develop a personalised, multifaceted treatment plan, remember that you don't have to do it alone. This part of the journey is the most challenging but also the most important, so it is worth spending some time to make it clear in your mind. Talk it through with a family member, friend or health professional if you are not sure how to develop your treatment plan.

In the next chapter, we'll explore practical steps to take with your chosen approach and identify the support systems you can rely on along the way.

It's time to take the first step towards reclaiming control of your life.

CHAPTER 8

Start Walking

The Road to Better Health

We've all heard the well-known Chinese proverb, 'A journey of a thousand miles begins with a single step.' While it's often used as a cliché to signify the start of a challenging process, the original quote, attributed to the Ancient Chinese philosopher Laozi (not Confucius), offers a slightly different perspective. A more literal translation reads, 'A journey of a thousand miles starts from where you stand.' This profound insight, first recorded around 500 BC, carries even greater weight when you consider the context of the time. Back then, embarking on a journey of a thousand miles – equivalent to roughly two million steps by some estimates – was fraught with uncertainty and risk, far removed from the conveniences of modern travel.

Now, imagine yourself in 500 BC, standing at the edge of your small village. There are no modern walking shoes, only simple sandals. Before you lies a long, dusty, winding path stretching into the unknown. Your future is uncertain, and the journey ahead is filled with both promise and challenge. This is where you stand now, ready to take that first step into a new exploration. To succeed, you'll need a sense of adventure, the courage to embrace both failure and success, and the resilience to navigate an uncharted path. While you may not know exactly where the road will lead, one thing is certain: it will take you somewhere new, somewhere better than where you've been before.

So, take that first step – your journey begins now.

Time To Start

You've now completed the five-step action plan and learned how to apply the biopsychosocial (BPS) model to your own life, helping you establish your starting point – your 'where you stand'. Now, it's time to take the next step: choosing your first intervention.

Perhaps addressing your poor sleep patterns feels like the easiest and most achievable starting point. Or maybe improving your diet has been on your mind for a while, and you've decided it's the right time to make that change. Whatever you've identified as your priority, the key is to begin implementing your action plan with a clear and deliberate first step.

Before you take that step, keep two crucial points in mind.

First, your initial intervention doesn't need to be an immediate dramatic game changer for your migraine disability. Small, consistent changes can still have a meaningful impact over time.

Second, regardless of how your migraine episodes respond in the short term, you are improving your overall health and wellbeing. Every positive change you make is a step towards a healthier, more balanced life.

Whatever you've chosen as your first intervention, it's time to delve deeper into how you'll approach this challenge. Empowering yourself with knowledge and building a support crew are essential steps to help you navigate this process successfully. Think of this chapter as your guidebook, designed to help you lift your foot and take that first step forward with confidence.

Interventions To Consider

The following pages provide a concise recap of the science behind each intervention and outline a game plan tailored to that specific treatment approach. You'll also gain a clear understanding of realistic timelines for improvement and learn who could be valuable members of your support crew for this stage of your journey. This may include expert health professionals where appropriate. Over time, you might find it beneficial to develop a multidisciplinary team rather than relying on a single expert to oversee everything.

Will this cover every possible approach or provide a detailed, step-by-step plan for the daily realities of each intervention? No, but it's a starting point. A game plan is just that – a plan – and it's natural for plans to evolve as you progress. The goal here is to reduce any sense of overwhelm and give you a clear, actionable place to begin. That's the purpose of this guide.

Please note that if you're feeling overwhelmed, it might be wise to go directly to your first two chosen interventions and review them to ensure you're comfortable with your decisions. Diving into all the interventions at once could lead to information overload, so focus on what's most relevant to you right now. Start small, stay focused and take it one step at a time.

The interventions listed are not in any particular order of importance.

Diet

A Quick Recap

The gut and brain are intricately connected through inflammatory-promoting chemicals and neurotransmitters carried in the bloodstream, as well as neurologically via the vagus nerve – one of the key cranial nerves that exits from the brainstem. This powerful, two-way relationship is known as the gut-brain axis.

A healthy gut plays a pivotal role in supporting a healthy brain. It contributes to improved energy levels, reduced inflammation and histamine production, and enhanced neurotransmitter production. Your diet is a key driver of these factors, significantly influencing brain health and helping to reduce the disability caused by migraine disease.

Diets high in carbohydrates, sugar and unhealthy fats, often found in processed and fast foods, can exacerbate inflammatory processes and histamine intolerance. Unfortunately, these foods are often the go-to choices for individuals fatigued and overwhelmed by the burden of migraine disability. However, these options can leave the brain and body undernourished, as the brain's energy demands are higher than normal due to its overactive state.

Making dietary improvements can also support the balanced functioning of the autonomic nervous system (ANS). Through the gut-brain axis, a healthier diet can help the brain resist excessive activation of the sympathetic nervous system (SNS) and reduce the impact of stress, which in turn helps to calm the sensitisation processes in the brain.

It's clear that your diet has the power to influence both your migraine and overall health in profound ways, either positively or negatively. By prioritising a nutrient-rich, balanced diet, you can take meaningful steps towards reducing migraine disability and improving your overall wellbeing.

What's the Game Plan?

Take a moment to evaluate your current knowledge of diet and nutrition. If you feel ready and have the mental space, consider doing some research to deepen your understanding and support informed decision-making.

When it comes to dietary changes, a gradual approach can often be beneficial. Personally, I found that making small, incremental changes over time allowed my body and brain to adapt more comfortably. However, a dietitian may recommend more significant adjustments to address your specific dietary needs or health goals.

It's important to remember that your sensitive migraine brain may not respond well to sudden, drastic changes in your fuel sources, potentially leading to an increase in migraine symptoms. If you're working with a dietitian, be sure to discuss this concern with them to ensure the approach aligns with your individual needs. Whether or not you're consulting a professional, it's essential to regularly assess how your body is responding to dietary changes. This process is highly individual, so take stock of your progress and adjust as needed to find what works best for you.

Here are some aspects of your diet which may prove useful to review.

Switch to Whole Foods

Transitioning to whole, unprocessed foods can have a profound impact on your gut health, which in turn supports brain health. Fresh, nutrient-dense foods are key, as opposed to heavily processed options. While this advice may sound familiar, the fibre and nutrients provided by whole foods make a significant difference to your gut microbiome. Foods like fresh fruits and vegetables, whole grains, nuts, lean meats and fish are staples often recommended by dietitians. These foods not only nourish your body but also help shift your energy sources towards protein and healthy fats, while reducing reliance on carbohydrates and sugars.

For example, salad leaves are a fantastic addition to your diet. They are rich in fibre and magnesium, which is essential for blocking the sensitising effects of calcium on nerves.[1] Magnesium, along with other nutrients like vitamin B1, B2 and zinc, is often lacking in western diets.[2] Incorporating these foods can help address these deficiencies and support overall health.

Eat the Rainbow

A simple and effective approach to improving your diet is to 'eat the rainbow'. This means including a variety of colours on your plate, especially when preparing salads. For instance, a vibrant salad might include a mix of salad leaves, capsicum, corn, beetroot, red onions, carrots and seeds. Adding a handful of berries, such as blueberries or raspberries, not only enhances the flavour but also provides essential vitamins while reducing the need for processed salad dressings. As an old friend once said, "There are no rules with a salad." The key is variety and balance.

Think About Supplements

Supplements should complement a healthy diet, not replace it. While the goal is to meet most of your nutritional needs through food, certain vitamins and trace elements may require supplementation. For example, vitamin B1, B2, magnesium and zinc are often beneficial for individuals with migraine disease. Omega-3 fatty acids, commonly found in fish oil, are another valuable supplement. While their role in reducing vascular disease has been debated, they remain highly effective for brain health and migraine management. Omega-3s have been shown to help regulate pain,[3] reduce stress, improve sleep and decrease migraine-related disability.[4] By targeting multiple factors associated with migraine, omega-3s can be a powerful addition to your treatment plan.

Creatine is another supplement worth considering. Known for its role in energy production, creatine is often used by athletes to support muscle recovery. For individuals with migraine, creatine may help boost energy levels in the brain, which can be particularly beneficial for managing migraine symptoms.

Additionally, there are specialised migraine supplements that combine essential vitamins and trace elements. For example, BioCeuticals Migraine Care includes B vitamins (B2 and B6), magnesium and co-enzyme Q10. These supplements aim to support neurotransmitter synthesis, nervous system function and energy production, while promoting a healthy stress response.

Consider Probiotics

If you suspect your gut microbiome could use some support, probiotics may be a helpful addition. Research has shown that probiotics, when used over a 10-week period, can significantly reduce the frequency and intensity of migraine episodes in individuals with episodic or chronic migraine.[5]

To maximise the benefits, consider rotating the types of probiotics you take. This variety ensures your gut receives a diverse range of beneficial bacteria, which can enhance its ability to break down food and provide the nutrients your body and brain need to function optimally.

Be Persistent

Making dietary changes is not always easy, and it's normal to encounter challenges along the way. Breaking old habits takes time, but persistence pays off. Over time, your tastes can adapt, and you may find surprising changes in your preferences. For instance, many people report a reduced craving for sugary foods and a newfound appreciation for savoury flavours as they adjust to a healthier diet.

By focusing on small, sustainable changes and staying consistent, you can create a diet that supports both your gut and brain health, ultimately helping to manage your migraine episodes and improve your overall wellbeing.

What's the Timeline?

Managing migraine through dietary changes is a long-term commitment. Think of it as a marathon, not a sprint. Progress may be slow at first, so it's important to set realistic expectations and be patient with yourself. Keeping a diary or journal to track your progress can be incredibly helpful. Document the dietary changes you make and note how they impact your symptoms. Over time, this record will provide valuable insights into what works best for you and help you stay motivated.

Who Can Help?

Navigating dietary changes for migraine is a specialised area that benefits greatly from professional guidance. Consulting a dietitian with expertise in migraine disease is highly recommended. Consultant migraine dietitian Thomas Paavola has extensive knowledge of migraine disease and understands the unique needs of the migraine brain. For instance, the migraine brain often struggles with energy efficiency, requiring more calories and a tailored approach to processing those calories into usable energy.

Paavola typically recommends a series of blood tests to identify nutrient and mineral deficiencies that can be addressed through a personalised nutrition program. This targeted approach is crucial, as incorrect dietary choices can exacerbate migraine. For example, sodium levels are often low in individuals with migraine. In such cases, Paavola may advise increasing salt intake, sometimes through drinking salty water, to address this deficiency. However, it's important to note that this advice is specific to individuals diagnosed with a sodium deficiency by a health professional. Generalised claims, such as those made by some social media influencers, should be approached with caution. If a claim sounds too good to be true, it likely is. Always rely on evidence-based advice from qualified professionals.

Your family can also play a significant role in supporting your dietary changes as their support may be essential for your success. Discuss your goals with your household, as dietary changes will inevitably affect everyone you eat with regularly, including your partner and children. Having their understanding and cooperation can make the process much smoother and more sustainable.

Additionally, following reputable social media accounts can provide ongoing education and motivation. For example, dietitian Kelli Yates offers regular scientific updates and positive reinforcement on her The Migraine Dietitian Instagram account, helping you stay informed and encouraged on your journey. Reliable resources like this can be a valuable tool in maintaining your commitment to dietary changes.

Stress

A Quick Recap

The ANS often operates in a state of dysfunction in individuals experiencing migraine. Specifically, the sympathetic part of the system becomes overactive, a condition commonly referred to as 'sympathetic overdrive'[6]. This response is typically triggered by three types of stress:

- **Lifestyle or Extrinsic Stress:** Daily pressures such as work demands, family responsibilities, and tight deadlines can create a constant state of urgency, leaving little time for relaxation and recovery. This type of stress is particularly prevalent in individuals aged 30 to 45 years, a demographic that often experiences the most significant life impact from migraine.

- **Adverse Childhood Events (ACEs) or Major Stressful Events:** An adverse childhood event can act as a precursor to migraine development in younger years. Similarly, any major stressful event later in life can push the ANS into a state of sympathetic overdrive, setting the stage for chronic migraine issues.

- **Intrinsic Migraine Stress:** The constant fear of an attack and its potential impact on daily life can create a persistent sense of vulnerability or feeling 'unsafe', leading to a hidden psychological burden. This stress is often exacerbated when friends and family fail to understand the condition's effects. The resulting loss of social interaction can further heighten pain levels and emotional distress, as is commonly observed in chronic pain conditions.[7]

While these factors may seem overwhelming, it's important to approach them step by step. Start with small, manageable changes and seek professional guidance. With the support of family and friends, you can navigate these challenges and find a path forward. Remember, progress is a journey, and every step counts!

What's the Game Plan?

Seeking the guidance of a psychologist can be a valuable step in managing stress and its impact on migraine. A psychologist can help you address both intrinsic and extrinsic stressors, as well as explore any significant past or recent stressful events that may have contributed to your migraine journey. Some experts argue that this aspect of stress management is often overlooked in the context of migraine.[8]

Working with a psychologist can help you develop strategies to calm your nervous system and reduce brainstem sensitivity. These sessions provide valuable tools to manage stress more effectively, minimising negative responses and promoting healthier coping mechanisms. A psychologist can support you by addressing past or present trauma, identifying psychological issues and managing ongoing concerns such as depression or anxiety. Additionally, they can teach practical and effective techniques to better manage and respond to stress in your daily life.

Improving the function of your ANS, particularly by calming the SNS, can significantly reduce stress and its effects. Here are some effective interventions you can explore yourself:

Mindfulness and Meditation

Mindfulness and meditation techniques can help you remain present during stressful situations, allowing you to stay calm and avoid 'wiring up', which can increase sensitisation. Regular practise of these techniques can have a profound calming effect on the nervous system.

Slow Deep Breathing and Relaxation Exercises

Slow, deep-breathing exercises stimulate the vagus nerve, activating the parasympathetic (relaxing) part of the ANS. Aim to reduce your breathing rate to four to six breaths per minute for optimal results. Yoga and stretching exercises, especially when combined with slow breathing, are also excellent tools for calming the nervous system.

Cold-Water Exposure

Although it may seem counterintuitive, cold-water exposure can have a calming effect on the nervous system. This can include cool to cold showers, winter swimming (if suitable for your location) or simply splashing cold water on your face. It's important to start at a comfortable level of cold and gradually reduce the water temperature over time. The goal is to calm the nervous system, not to stress it further, so extreme measures like ice baths are unnecessary.

Social Interaction

Planning social activities to maintain relationships with friends and family is an effective way to de-stress and calm your ANS. Try to plan your social activities in a way that maintains your sense of safety. This will include choosing an appropriate venue with minimal sensory load and feeling comfortable to cancel if a migraine episode disrupts your plans.

Spending Time in Nature

Time in nature is a simple yet powerful way to calm the nervous system. Activities such as swimming in natural water environments or walking in the bush can work wonders. Many people have a preferred option – where I live in Cronulla, Sydney, we are fortunate to have access to both. The stunning beaches and the Royal National Park offer the perfect settings for relaxation. Personally, I enjoy mountain biking through the National Park with a mate on Saturday mornings, followed by a refreshing beach swim. Combining exercise, nature and social interaction in this way ticks multiple boxes for stress relief.

Improving Sleep

If stress is affecting your sleep, which is common, focusing on sleep hygiene can be a helpful follow-up to mindfulness and relaxation techniques. Quality sleep is essential for overall wellbeing and can further support your efforts to calm the ANS.

By incorporating these strategies into your routine, you can take meaningful steps towards managing stress and improving your overall health. Remember, progress takes time, so start small and build gradually. With professional guidance and support from loved ones, you can create a sustainable path to better wellbeing.

What's the Timeline?

The timeline for seeing results from mindfulness and relaxation techniques is highly individual and depends on several factors, including the areas of stress affected, your life circumstances and the support systems available to you. If you start by learning practical techniques to de-stress, you may notice benefits relatively quickly, often within a few weeks.

However, if you are addressing deeper psychological challenges, the process may take longer. In such cases, it's realistic to expect at least three to six months before you begin to see significant results. Remember, this is likely to be an ongoing journey, but the rewards, such as reduced migraine attacks and improved overall wellbeing, are invaluable. Patience and consistency are key, as the long-term benefits will far outweigh the effort invested.

Who Can Help?

A trusted psychologist is an essential part of your support system when addressing stress and its impact on your health. Their expertise can guide you through the process of understanding and managing stress effectively.

In addition to professional help, don't underestimate the value of support from friends and family, especially your partner if you have one. Consider asking one or more people to be part of your support team. Be specific about the kind of help you need – whether it's a listening ear, practical assistance or simply someone to check in on you regularly. Clear communication about your needs can make a significant difference in the support you receive.

While social media should be approached with caution in the realm of health advice, some resources can be insightful. For example, Dr Nicole LePera's Instagram account The Holistic Psychologist offers thought-provoking content that may resonate with you.

Additionally, the S.A.F.E.T.Y.™ domains explained by Leonie Hull in Chapter 6 provide valuable insights into understanding your stress responses and how to navigate them effectively.[9]

By combining professional guidance, personal support and evidence-based resources, you can create a strong foundation for managing stress and improving your health.

Upper Neck Dysfunction

A Quick Recap

The neck plays a significant role in migraine across all age groups. In infants, migraine has been linked to acute torticollis, a condition involving neck tightness and muscle spasm. This connection persists into adolescence and adulthood, where neck pain is often associated with migraine. Furthermore, research has linked neck involvement to the chronification of migraine, where the frequency of migraine days increases to at least eight days per month. It is also linked to greater disability, reduced quality of life and higher rates of lost productivity at work.

The reason for this strong association potentially lies in the neurological connection between the upper neck and the brainstem. The nerves of the top three vertebrae in the neck, along with those associated with the muscles of the occipital triangle at the base of the skull, have direct links to the brainstem. These nerves also connect to the amygdala and the ANS, which are critical in regulating stress responses and pain perception.

Many patients report a clear connection between their neck and migraine episodes, often describing neck pain or stiffness as a precursor or accompanying symptom. However, there remains some hesitancy within the medical community to fully acknowledge this association. This reluctance may stem from a lack of understanding of how dysfunction in the upper neck can disrupt brainstem sensitivity.

Despite this uncertainty, it is essential not to overlook the neck when assessing migraine or headaches. Just as migraine can mimic other headache types, other headache types can present similarly to migraine. A thorough evaluation of the neck can provide valuable insights and may help guide treatment strategies for those experiencing migraine.

The Watson Headache® Approach (WHA) is a manual therapy technique that applies gentle, sustained pressure to reproduce familiar headache pain. Over a decade ago, this method was shown to influence brainstem sensitivity, a key factor in migraine. More recently, a similar technique that did not reproduce familiar headache pain also demonstrated a reduction in brainstem sensitivity. This suggests that other sustained manual therapy techniques may have a similar effect. A recent review also revealed a variety of neck treatment interventions that yielded positive results for individuals with migraine.[10]

What's the Game Plan?

Consider your options for manual therapy with a physiotherapist. You may wish to start by trying the WHA, which is designed to address upper neck dysfunction and its relevance to migraine within a short timeframe – typically four to five treatments over two to four weeks, depending on individual circumstances. During this period, the goal is to identify the presence of upper neck dysfunction and its connection to migraine symptoms. Ideally, patients will experience some improvement or a noticeable change in their migraine presentation, indicating a positive influence on their attacks. Achieving optimal results with the WHA may take longer, as the approach aims to retrain the brain to avoid entering 'migraine mode'.

Additionally, complementary treatments can enhance the effectiveness of the WHA. For example, strengthening exercises for the neck, particularly targeting the deep neck flexors, can improve muscle support and reduce the likelihood of upper neck dysfunction. Joint position error (JPE) testing is another valuable tool, as it assesses and improves muscle control patterns in the neck. When neck muscles function efficiently, the risk of brainstem sensitisation decreases.

If you experience dizziness as a migraine symptom, consider a vestibular assessment. These assessments help identify the causes of dizziness and contribute to brainstem desensitisation through the principle of exposure. By gradually challenging the nerves with specific sensations, they can become less reactive over time. However, it is crucial to ensure that the exposure is not too intense, as this could exacerbate symptoms.

Manual therapy for the upper neck can also be effectively combined with other treatments, such as Botox. Botox is a muscle-relaxing agent used in migraine treatment, administered in small doses at multiple sites in the head and neck. Anecdotal evidence from collaborations with neurologists at Southern Neurology suggests that combining Botox with the WHA can be a powerful approach to managing migraine.

By integrating manual therapy, strengthening exercises, vestibular assessments and complementary treatments like Botox, individuals experiencing migraine can benefit from a comprehensive and tailored approach to managing their symptoms.

What's the Timeline?

One of the advantages of the WHA is that it does not require a long-term commitment to weekly treatments, which is often the case with other approaches. The WHA typically takes three to four weeks to assess whether there has been any meaningful change in your migraine symptoms. Establishing a more consistent and lasting change may take two to three months, accounting for normal weekly or monthly variations in symptoms. Compared to many other migraine interventions, this is a relatively short timeframe. Observing noticeable changes within just a few weeks can provide a significant psychological boost for individuals navigating the challenges of a long migraine journey.

Who Can Help?

It's highly recommended to seek out a practitioner experienced in the WHA, as it is a proven method for addressing upper neck dysfunction and its connection to migraine – the practitioner directory at www.watsonheadache.com is helpful for this. If finding a WHA practitioner is not possible, other sustained manual therapy techniques, such as Mulligan techniques, may also be beneficial. Ultimately, the effectiveness of any treatment will depend on your individual experience and response, so it's important to evaluate whether a particular approach is worth continuing.

Additionally, you could also consider seeking recommendations for physiotherapists who have a special interest in treating headaches. When consulting with a physiotherapist, ask about their approach to treating upper neck dysfunction and how their treatment plans are structured. Each practitioner's methods may vary slightly, but your primary goal should be to find someone who understands the complexities of migraine as a neurological condition. This understanding will give you the best chance of determining whether upper neck dysfunction is contributing to your migraine symptoms.

A skilled therapist can also guide you through a tailored strength program and provide advice on improving your posture, which can complement upper neck treatments. They will recognise the importance of exercise, whether it's aerobic training or weightlifting, as a potential pathway to improvement. However, they will also understand that high-intensity exercise or lifting very heavy weights may trigger neck issues and potentially exacerbate your migraine presentation. A knowledgeable therapist will help you select the most appropriate exercises to support your recovery and minimise the risk of aggravating your symptoms.

Sleep

A Quick Recap

High-quality sleep is crucial for overall health but can be particularly challenging for individuals who experience migraine. This is due to shared dysfunctional brain pathways, neuro-inflammation, comorbidities and poor long-term sleep habits often established in childhood.

Medication is often the first intervention, with melatonin becoming increasingly popular. However, responses to melatonin can vary. A 2017 research paper revealed that many melatonin supplements contain levels that differ significantly from what is stated on the packaging,[11] which may explain some of these inconsistent results.

The benefits of a consistent and effective sleep pattern are immense, as restorative sleep is both essential and transformative. However, maintaining a regular sleep schedule can be difficult, as it requires going to bed and waking up at the same time every day, including weekends. Life's unpredictable events, such as welcoming a new baby, can disrupt this routine, potentially leading to more frequent migraine episodes. If poor sleep patterns persist, it can take time to re-establish healthier habits. For those who have struggled with sleep for a long time, the brain must relearn the process.

Although it takes time, with better sleep the brain will benefit from improved glymphatic drainage, which clears waste products, reduces inflammation and enhances immune responses. These improvements can lower brainstem sensitivity, reducing your likelihood of reaching the migraine threshold.

What's the Game Plan?

Sleep specialists often recommend natural methods, particularly for chronic sleep deprivation. The goal is to re-establish a consistent sleep pattern, and there are several strategies to try:

Develop a Regular Sleep Cycle

Go to bed and wake up at the same time every day. Use your bed only for sleep – avoid watching television, using social media, eating or reading in bed. Train your brain to associate your bed with sleep.

Find Your Comfort Zone

Keep your bedroom cool (but not cold) for an optimal sleep environment. Ensure the room is dark and quiet and have extra blankets within reach to avoid disruptions during the night.

Establish Daily Habits to Help You Sleep at Night

Get early morning sunlight to regulate your sleep–wake cycle. Stay active during the day through exercise or other activities to promote recovery and induce sleep hormones. Avoid napping during the day unless you are unwell. Limit caffeine intake after midday, as it blocks adenosine, a chemical that promotes sleep. In the evening, reduce light exposure by using dimmer switches and avoid blue light from screens at least one to two hours before bedtime. Incorporate relaxing activities such as yoga, stretching, deep breathing or meditation into your pre-sleep routine to prepare your body and mind for restful sleep.

Once you've established boundaries and a framework for your sleep patterns, learning relaxation techniques can be a valuable next step.

What's the Timeline?

Defining a timeline for improved sleep is challenging, as sleep should be viewed as an ongoing priority. Research underscores the importance of sleep, which, unlike exercise, is non-negotiable for survival. The goal is to find a sleep pattern that works for you and maintain it. Life events will inevitably disrupt these patterns, but the key is to re-establish them as quickly as possible.

Who Can Help?

Sleep studies and specialist support may be beneficial, and these options can be discussed with your doctor. Many natural methods for improving sleep patterns are available that do not require medications. Remember your brain has, most likely, 'learned' poor sleep patterns from an early age so it will be a process to learn new and more restorative processes. As is the case with many of these interventions, you are teaching your brain a new skill – be patient and expect some good and bad days through the process.

Ensure that any information you rely on is from reputable sources. A sleep specialist or your doctor can guide you in the right direction. If a young family is affecting your sleep quality, consider seeking help from a family member or friend to share the load.

Exercise

A Quick Recap

The role of exercise in maintaining health is widely acknowledged, and the type of exercise required often depends on the condition being addressed. For migraine, which involves both neurological and vascular components, exercises that influence these areas can be particularly beneficial.

Research has found that moderate-intensity aerobic exercise and yoga are highly effective in reducing the frequency, intensity and duration of migraine attacks while also improving overall quality of life. Other forms of exercise, such as high-intensity interval training (HIIT), continuous low-intensity exercise, Tai Chi and strength training, have shown moderate effectiveness.

Aerobic exercise offers additional benefits that indirectly impact migraine management. These include improved sleep quality, enhanced cardiovascular efficiency, reduced inflammation and a more positive psychological outlook.[12,13] It also supports general health by reducing obesity and lowering the risk of heart attacks and strokes, which are known comorbidities of migraine. Interestingly, some studies suggest that reduced obesity may enhance the effectiveness of migraine-specific medications.[14] For instance, recent research indicates that individuals who walked regularly before starting newer medications experienced better outcomes than those who were sedentary.[15] These wide-ranging benefits make aerobic exercise one of the most appealing interventions for migraine management.

Incorporating physical activity into your migraine management plan can be transformative. The specifics of your exercise routine can be tailored to your personal circumstances and preferences within a structured framework.

What's the Game Plan?

Your choice of exercise protocol should align with your personal preferences, existing health conditions, family medical history, age and lifestyle. Here are some general guidelines to help you decide where to start:

Get off the Couch

If migraine has kept you sedentary, the key question to ask yourself is: what will inspire me to start moving? Forcing yourself into an activity you dislike is unlikely to be effective. Instead, consider an activity – let's not call it exercise just yet – that you might genuinely enjoy. Walking is a great option but think about enhancing the experience: perhaps a stroll by the water, through a park or in bushland with a scenic view. You could even turn it into a social activity by walking with a friend – an active catch-up followed by a coffee. Often, it's the idea of a traditional 'workout' that feels overwhelming or discouraging, so reframing it as something enjoyable and manageable can make all the difference.

If you've been relatively active, setting a goal can help guide your efforts. For example, I signed up to do an endurance event called the Spartan Race which provided an extra challenge to help me focus on my training. I also involved a few friends in my fitness journey, which served as a powerful motivator.

Aerobic Exercise

This form of exercise is highly recommended due to its extensive benefits for brain health, psychological wellbeing and overall health. If a full aerobic program (e.g. 30 minutes, three to four times per week) feels overwhelming, consider alternatives like yoga or Tai Chi. These activities can reduce stress, improve strength and flexibility, and require less time and physical strain.

For aerobic exercise parameters, aim for moderate intensity – 30 minutes of activity that raises your heart rate (HR) to 64–76% of your maximum. To calculate your maximum HR, subtract your age from 220. For example, if you're 35 years old, your maximum HR is 185, and your target range for moderate exercise is 118–140 beats per minute.

If you've been sedentary, start with low-intensity exercise, which is 50–63% of your maximum HR. For a 35-year-old, this would be 92–118 beats per minute. A brisk walk with a friend can make this more enjoyable and achievable.

Building Motivation

For those lacking motivation, start with any activity that gets you moving. Yoga is a great option – begin with a beginner's class or private lessons to build confidence.

Strength Training

Strength training can be beneficial, even if you're unsure about your muscle strength. Focus on light weights, proper technique, functional movements and high repetitions to build confidence and prepare your body for more intense activity.

Be Careful

If you haven't exercised regularly in years, avoid HIIT training initially, as it can lead to injuries. If exercise triggers your migraine episodes, be careful to progress your intensity levels slowly. Give your body time to adjust to the new activity levels that your migraine brain can react to in a negative way. A negative reaction may also indicate stress on your upper neck, so seek treatment for your neck and consider complementary strategies like improving sleep patterns or practising relaxation techniques.

What's the Timeline?

For aerobic exercise, research suggests that noticeable changes in migraine patterns can occur within three months of reaching the required intensity.[16,17] For other forms of exercise, such as yoga or strength training, evidence is less definitive. Psychological benefits may appear within weeks, but physical changes typically take two to three months.

Who Can Help?

A personal trainer can help you get started and stay on track. Be clear about your goals and how they relate to your migraine attacks. If you have multiple health concerns, an exercise physiologist with advanced training in illness-related exercise may be ideal. A physiotherapist can assist if migraine or other injuries are affecting your ability to exercise.

An exercise partner can also provide motivation and support. A long walk with a friend can double as both physical activity and psychological encouragement.

Trigger Management

A Quick Recap

Managing triggers requires time and careful analysis; however, it can be valuable, especially if you suspect certain triggers are contributing to your migraine episodes yet cannot pinpoint the exact factors.

Common triggers include neck pain (43%), tiredness (33%) and restless sleep (25%). Environmental triggers such as smells/odours, bright lights and loud noise are all prevalent in the mid-20% range. Weather plays a role, with high temperatures (32%) and high humidity (17%) being common triggers, while changes in barometric pressure are less frequent (4%). Food triggers and physical activity each have a lower impact (2–4%).[18] Many of these triggers directly affect nonconscious regions of the brain neurologically.

The terms 'trigger' and 'factor' are often used interchangeably when discussing migraine. Research suggests that most individuals have up to four triggers, although some may have as many as 10. It's important to understand that each person's trigger profile is unique. While the most recent or most noticeable factor is often labelled as the 'trigger' for a migraine, it's essential to recognise that all contributing factors collectively play a role in the migraine process. Identifying your specific contributing factors allows for more effective management.

What's the Game Plan?

The N1-Headache app is an excellent tool for this approach. Unlike a standard migraine diary, which only records potential triggers around migraine episodes, the N1-Headache app tracks the presence or absence of 33 major triggers daily for 90 days. This comprehensive analysis not only identifies your triggers but also reveals how they interact to cause a migraine episode.

While there is a cost to the app and a demand on your time for 90 days, there could be significant benefits to the process. Remember it is akin to trying to separate cake ingredients after the cake has been baked – it's going to be a tough road to walk for a season, but it will most likely smooth out the path for the future.

One key challenge during the 90-day recording process is resisting the urge to eliminate suspected triggers prematurely. It's crucial to maintain your usual habits during this period, as the goal is to identify whether a trigger acts independently or in combination with others. For instance, you might find that consuming cheese and alcohol together on hot days is a powerful trigger for a migraine attack, whereas eating cheese or drinking alcohol alone has no effect. Without this insight, you could be avoiding cheese unnecessarily, when in reality, it's only problematic in specific circumstances – such as when combined with alcohol on hot days.

Understanding specific triggers can also lead to targeted interventions. For instance, if hot weather is a trigger and you live in a warm climate, strategies like drinking more water or staying indoors during peak heat could help reduce migraine episodes. Or, if you plan to attend a concert with bright lights and loud noise (known triggers), you can prepare by ensuring you are well rested, eating clean, practising relaxation techniques and staying hydrated. These steps can help lower your brainstem sensitivity and reduce the likelihood of a migraine episode spoiling your night out.

What's the Timeline?

To gather reliable data, you'll need to use the tracking app consistently for three months before making any changes. Keep in mind that other interventions, such as medications or strategies previously discussed, may positively influence your list of triggers.

Although this process may feel lengthy, it is particularly beneficial for complex migraine presentations that are difficult to analyse. A scientific and methodical approach can provide much-needed clarity. Additionally, understanding your migraine triggers can reduce stress and improve your overall quality of life.

Who Can Help?

Gaining a deeper understanding of your triggers can open up new management possibilities. For example, if dietary triggers are significant, consulting a dietitian would be a logical next step. If sleep issues are a major factor, seeking advice from a sleep specialist may be beneficial.

While a support person is less critical for this task, as most of the work involves your own diligent recording of triggers, having a friend to discuss your findings with can be helpful. Recording triggers can be labour-intensive, so emotional support and encouragement may make the process more manageable.

Medication Overuse Headache (MOH)

A Quick Recap

Migraine is the most common headache type associated with the development of medication overuse headache (MOH), accounting for 80% of all such cases. MOH often arises when migraine progresses from episodic to chronic due to the frequent use of basic analgesics, triptans or codeine-based medications over a three-month period.[19] This progression is likely linked to the intensity of migraine symptoms, as many individuals find it difficult to endure the severe pain of a migraine attack without seeking relief through medication.

If MOH is present, the benefits of medication withdrawal are significant. Reducing medication use often decreases migraine frequency, potentially shifting a person from a chronic migraine classification to an episodic one. Research suggests that reducing medication in MOH cases can influence epigenetic factors, leading to a decrease in neuro-inflammatory chemicals in the brain[20] and improvements in gut health.[21] These changes collectively reduce overall brain sensitivity, particularly in the brainstem, thereby lowering the risk of migraine attacks.

This is where a multifaceted treatment approach can create a synergistic effect. Enhancing diet and addressing MOH can both contribute to improved gut health, which in turn positively impacts brain health.

What's the Game Plan?

If you are considering reducing your medication usage, it is essential to seek medical advice before starting the process. A healthcare professional can confirm whether you are indeed overusing medication, as some individuals avoid taking any medication out of concern for MOH, potentially missing out on the benefits of effective pain relief. Given the complexity of MOH, working with a neurologist or general practitioner to develop a tailored medication plan is highly recommended.

If MOH is identified as an issue, there are two primary approaches to reducing medication use:

- **Cold turkey:** involves completely stopping the medication. This method is generally suitable for simple analgesics or triptan medications that are purchased over the counter.
- **Gradual reduction:** medication use is slowly decreased over time. This method is particularly recommended for codeine-based medications, as abruptly stopping these can lead to significant side effects.

Regardless of the method chosen, education is crucial. Studies have shown that education improves outcomes and helps establish effective results.[22,23] While there is no universal consensus on the best approach to reducing overused medication, a personalised program that considers your medical history and social circumstances (BPS approach) is considered the most effective.[23]

A newer strategy involves the use of 'bridge therapy' to support the weaning process. This includes incorporating an additional treatment to help manage the transition away from medication reliance. For example, mindfulness programs have been shown to benefit some individuals with

MOH.[24] Other potential interventions, such as aerobic exercise or upper neck treatment, may also help by calming brainstem sensitivity and supporting the medication reduction process. These secondary interventions can be introduced after the initial phase of medication reduction has stabilised.

What's the Timeline?

Research indicates that a two-month program is typically required to achieve positive long-term results, even in chronic MOH cases.[22] This makes it a particularly valuable intervention for those feeling overwhelmed by the relentless challenges of living with migraine. By offering the potential for relatively quick improvements, this approach can provide a much-needed morale boost, especially if your journey with migraine has felt like navigating an uneven and steep trail. The prospect of regaining some control and seeing tangible progress within a short timeframe can be incredibly empowering, serving as a stepping stone towards a healthier, more balanced life.

Who Can Help?

Consulting a neurologist is highly beneficial as they are best qualified to create an effective medication plan. The primary goals are to reduce overused medications and establish appropriate parameters for their use. While creating a personalised medication plan may take time, it is a valuable investment in your long-term health.

Psychological support, including education and mindfulness programs, is also highly recommended. Building psychological resilience is beneficial not only for addressing medication overuse but also for overall migraine management and rehabilitation.

Hormonal Management (MOH)

A Quick Recap

Menstrual migraine affects approximately 6% of women in their reproductive years. It is characterised by the onset of migraine within two days before or after menstruation. In its pure form, menstrual migraine occurs exclusively during this time, and research indicates that it is often associated with higher pain intensity and more severe associated symptoms. Menstrual-related migraine, on the other hand, occurs during menstruation but can also arise at other times.

The long-standing 'oestrogen withdrawal hypothesis' suggests that fluctuating hormonal levels, particularly the drop in oestrogen, play a significant role in triggering a migraine attack. However, this relationship is not always straightforward. Factors such as genetics, hormonal variations and heightened brainstem sensitivity can all contribute to the onset of migraine episodes, making it a complex condition to define and manage.[25]

What's the Game Plan?

Effectively managing hormonal migraine requires a tailored approach. Research suggests that combining migraine-specific medications with hormonal treatments often yields better results than relying solely on migraine medications.[26]

Hormonal treatments for menstrual migraine range from minimally invasive options, such as birth control pills or hormonal injections, to more invasive procedures like a hysterectomy. However, the latter is a rare intervention, typically reserved for cases where all other options have been exhausted.

It's also important to address other factors that contribute to brainstem sensitivity, as this can help mitigate the impact of hormonal fluctuations. For instance, a 2015 pilot study found a link between neck dysfunction and menstrual migraine.[27] Addressing upper neck issues to reduce brainstem sensitivity may lessen the effects of oestrogen withdrawal on the migraine process. Similarly, incorporating exercise or mindfulness techniques could provide additional benefits.

If you're unsure about the role of hormonal changes in your migraine presentation, consider using the N1-Headache app to track your triggers over a three-month period. This can help you identify patterns and clarify how hormonal fluctuations interact with other triggers, reducing stress and providing valuable insights.

What's the Timeline?

Managing hormonal migraine can be particularly challenging, especially when hormonal changes are a primary trigger. Fortunately, it is uncommon for hormonal fluctuations to be the sole factor in migraine episodes. However, due to the ongoing nature of hormonal changes over time, it can be difficult to establish a consistent pattern or timeline for treatment. This is often an ongoing process that requires patience and adaptability.

Who Can Help?

A multidisciplinary approach is often necessary to effectively manage hormonal migraine. This may include support from gynaecologists, endocrinologists, psychologists and neurologists. If hormonal treatments alone are not providing relief, consider exploring other interventions discussed in this chapter. Additionally, having the support of a partner, family member or close friend can be invaluable in navigating the challenges of treatment and recovery.

Conclusion

The journey to managing migraine has begun, but the destination may still feel uncertain. This lack of clarity can be unsettling, as we naturally crave a defined goal and a clear roadmap to guide us. In 500 BC, our ancestors embarked on long journeys without maps or guides. Their travels were filled with ongoing decisions and adjustments. Similarly, your migraine journey will likely follow a comparable path, requiring patience and adaptability. Imagine yourself in your ancestors' shoes.

Migraine is as unique as the individuals who experience it. Even if you compare your experiences with someone who has a similar migraine pattern, you'll likely discover that your healing journeys differ significantly. Each path is personal, shaped by individual triggers, responses and circumstances. Embrace this uniqueness and remember that progress is not always linear – it's about finding what works best for you.

By now, you should understand that there is no quick fix for migraine. However, there are steps you can take to move forward and improve your quality of life. Think of a holistic approach to migraine management as an investment in a healthier, pain-reduced future.

As discussed, migraine is often influenced by a combination of genetic, lifestyle and environmental factors. This means that multiple interventions may be necessary to see meaningful change. It's also important to remember that progress takes time, especially given the natural variations in migraine patterns.

Consider the circular nature of these interventions. By adopting new ways of living, you can influence the way your neurological pathways function. The goal is to reduce the sensitivity and reactivity of these pathways. As they begin to function more efficiently, your life journey can feel safer, more stable, and ultimately, more fulfilling by your newfound knowledge.

If you haven't already, start journalling your process. A simple notebook can become an invaluable resource, allowing you to track your progress, reflect on your journey and identify patterns or triggers. This record will also guide your decisions about future interventions, helping you and your support team – whether family, friends or health professionals – make informed choices about the next steps.

Journalling also provides a tangible way to measure progress, even when it feels slow. It can emphasise the small victories that might otherwise go unnoticed and serve as a reminder of how far you've come.

Now, let's explore how this process of progression might unfold and how you can continue to build on the foundation you've started.

CHAPTER 9

Embracing Change

Moving Towards a Better Future

You've embarked on a long and transformative journey and taking that first step is often the hardest part. While you may have done some planning and preparation, it's natural not to see progress just yet. Unlike the convenience of modern navigation apps that guide us step by step, this journey doesn't come with a pre-mapped route.

Think of it as travelling in 500 BC – uncharted, unpredictable and requiring you to adapt as you go. At times, it may feel like you're simply trying to survive, but this is all part of the process. Adjustments and redirections will be necessary, and while they may feel challenging, they are essential to finding your way forward.

Embrace the idea of flexibility and resilience. Each step, even the uncertain ones, is a step closer to your goal. Progress may not always be visible, but it is happening. Trust in the process and remember that every small adjustment is a sign of growth and learning.

This journey is not about perfection; it's about persistence. Keep moving forward, one step at a time, and allow yourself the grace to adapt and evolve along the way.

Assessing your response to the first intervention is crucial before determining your next step. This reflective process ensures that each intervention builds on the last, creating a cumulative effect that drives meaningful and sustainable improvement.

Our goal is to foster progress through the combined impact of multiple interventions. To maintain motivation and avoid burnout, it's essential to break the journey into small, manageable steps – bite-sized actions that feel achievable and empowering.

From the previous chapter, you should have a few potential progressions for your second intervention. To help you decide on the next step, here are some practical tips:

- **Evaluate the impact of the first intervention:** Reflect on how the initial intervention has influenced your symptoms, lifestyle and overall wellbeing. Identify what worked well and what could be improved.
- **Set clear priorities:** Determine which area of your health or lifestyle you'd like to focus on next. Whether it's stress management, physical activity or dietary changes, choose a priority that aligns with your current needs and goals.
- **Start with manageable steps:** Select an intervention that feels realistic and achievable. Small, consistent changes are more likely to lead to long-term success without overwhelming you.
- **Seek professional guidance:** If you're unsure about the next step, consult a healthcare professional or trusted advisor to ensure your plan is evidence-based and tailored to your unique circumstances.
- **Stay adaptable:** Be open to adjusting your approach as you learn more about what works best for you. Flexibility is key to navigating challenges and maintaining progress.

By focusing on incremental progress and building on each intervention, you'll create a sustainable path towards improvement. Trust the process, celebrate small wins and remember that every step forward is a step closer to your goal.

Refining Your Path to the Next Intervention

Your next intervention naturally builds upon the foundation of your first choice, its level of success and your personal time constraints and motivation. Ideally, you've experienced at least a small win, giving you the confidence to move forward. If progress has been slower than expected, don't lose heart. Starting this journey is a significant step, and you've already made clear decisions about prioritising your health. Now, it's time to build on that groundwork.

Your next step might be as straightforward as revisiting your initial checklist and selecting the next intervention. Alternatively, your first intervention may have provided insights or clues that point to a logical next move. Revisiting Chapter 8 can offer a structured game plan to help you take that next step with clarity and purpose.

I want to reinforce that progressions are highly individualised. It's important to remember that no two migraine sufferers will follow the same path. You may find yourself with several potential 'next steps' and need to prioritise which to tackle first. Alternatively, you might discover that your chosen intervention doesn't align perfectly with your current lifestyle, requiring adjustments along the way. Flexibility and self-awareness are key.

By staying adaptable and focused, you can continue to make meaningful progress towards better health and wellbeing.

My Second Intervention

Discovering the Watson Headache® Approach (WHA) marked a turning point in managing my migraine. The treatment and neck exercises significantly improved my condition, though morning headaches and the fear of migraines returning lingered. Without access to WHA, I continued the exercises, sought conventional neck therapy and occasionally used codeine-based medications to manage pain.

Over the years, stress was a key trigger and I had a few close calls with migraines. One occurred during a nerve-wracking physiotherapy sports specialisation exam, where I battled a significant headache with borderline migraine symptoms. Another was at the 2016 NRL Grand Final, where my team, the Cronulla Sharks, won their first premiership after nearly 50 years. The stress-induced headache during the second half was intense, but I managed to stay for the thrilling finish. Ten years earlier, such stress would have triggered a full-blown migraine, leaving me unable to participate in the exam or enjoy the winning moment.

At age 48, I was facing high cholesterol and a weight of 83 kg. I made gradual lifestyle changes, motivated by my father's near-fatal heart attack. I replaced sugary foods with nutrient-rich meals, reduced processed foods and introduced supplements like magnesium and fish oil. While intermittent fasting wasn't suitable due to its potential to trigger migraines, consistent meal patterns and reduced sugar intake supported my migraine-prone brain.

These changes not only improved my overall health but also reduced my headache sensitivity. I went from frequent codeine use to rarely needing pain relief, and my cholesterol normalised. Now, at 63, I feel healthier than I did 15 years ago, with migraines reduced to just three mild episodes in 17 years. I no longer feel controlled by the condition, physically or mentally.

Keep Moving Forward

On this journey, progress might not always follow a straight path, but persistence remains essential.

Keep an eye on the bigger picture. Life changes, and so do the factors influencing your migraine presentation. By the time you reach your third intervention, your circumstances may look very different from when you started. Has a major life event caused significant stress? Has your neurologist adjusted your medications? These changes can influence how migraine behaves and may affect the effectiveness of your current intervention. If you're in the middle of a treatment, understand that it might take longer to see results due to these shifting conditions. If you're searching for your next step, these changes could provide valuable insights. Either way, maintaining a headache diary and tracking your progress over time is essential.

Take a moment to reflect on what you haven't yet explored.

What about exercise? You may have an aversion to being active but even minimal levels of exercise at a modest-intensity load can make a difference. The key is to find a pursuit you enjoy – an exercise partner can also make it more agreeable.

Could neck treatment be worth considering? Even if you don't have obvious neck symptoms, many people unknowingly adapt to limitations in their neck mobility. After treatment or exercises, patients often report newfound freedom of movement, realising they had simply adjusted to the restriction as their 'new normal'. Remember, the goal isn't just to address a musculoskeletal condition – it's to reduce brainstem sensitivity, which is a different approach than what you might expect from a typical physiotherapy consultation.

Consistency is one of the biggest challenges when trying new interventions. It's easier to stay consistent if you're also aiming to improve your overall health alongside managing migraine. Seek advice from your medical team and consider researching interventions to stay motivated. For example, research led me to explore other lifestyle changes that intrigued me. Over time, I adjusted my gym routine to include more high-intensity interval training (HIIT). Since HIIT can be physically demanding, I introduced it gradually to avoid overexertion. I also experimented with cold exposure through showers and winter swims, though I've avoided full immersion ice baths for now – they can be taxing on the body, but perhaps I'll try them in the future. Looking ahead, I'm considering exploring psychologically based programs like relaxation techniques or mindfulness.

There's no shortage of options to try, so don't give up! The journey requires commitment, resilience and a willingness to navigate ups and downs. If you've lived with migraine for any length of time, you're already familiar with this kind of perseverance.

It's important to acknowledge that our understanding of migraine as a disease is still evolving, and significant breakthroughs may not happen in the short to medium term.

Additionally, the healthcare resources available to you will depend on factors like your location and socioeconomic circumstances. Applying the biopsychosocial (BPS) model is inherently subjective, meaning no one can predict exactly how you, as an individual, will respond to a specific treatment. This variability applies not only to medications but also to lifestyle approaches.

The key takeaway? Keep moving forward. Stay open to new possibilities, track your progress and remain committed to the process.

Advocating for Yourself

Adjusting to a holistic model of migraine management takes time, patience and persistence. As your health improves, you'll build resilience and gain momentum in reversing the downward spiral of symptoms. This journey is not without its challenges, but with determination and the right support, you can make meaningful progress.

Leaning on family and friends can be a cornerstone of your success. Consider assembling a small support network to encourage and assist you along the way.

However, it's important to remember that this is *your* journey. The willpower to make changes must come from within. The adjustments you're making, whether to your lifestyle choices or brain pathways, are deeply personal. The benefits you'll gain will smooth the road ahead, making your life's journey more comfortable and fulfilling. Taking ownership of your health and advocating for the steps you believe are best is a vital part of this process.

The holistic approach to health is not a new concept. The BPS model, which integrates biological, psychological and social factors, has been a recommended pathway for better health for over 75 years. However, this approach often contrasts with traditional migraine treatments, so it's not uncommon to encounter resistance from your medical team.[1] If this happens, remind yourself – and your healthcare providers – of the goals you're striving to achieve through a holistic approach.

Goal 1: Long-Term Health Improvements

Your focus isn't solely on short-term relief from migraine symptoms. Instead, you're addressing your individual needs and aiming for disease prevention at multiple levels. This approach ensures that, regardless of the interventions you choose, you'll experience long-term health benefits, not just temporary symptom relief.

Goal 2: Breaking the Vicious Cycle

Migraine often creates a cycle where symptoms lead to further brainstem and central sensitisation, worsening the condition. By adopting a holistic approach, you're working to break this cycle and reduce the overall impact of migraine on your life.

Goal 3: Enhancing Quality of Life

Your ultimate goal is to improve your overall quality of life. Whether an intervention reduces social isolation, alleviates stress or lessens physical pain, any improvement is a step forward and validates the effort you've invested in trying something new.

When meeting with your medical team, bring your journal notes and clearly outline your health and migraine goals. This will help you communicate your progress and advocate for the holistic approach you're pursuing.

As you navigate this journey, stay focused and be kind to yourself. Avoid making too many changes at once, as this can lead to confusion about what is or isn't working. Your body and mind will respond better to a 'hurry slowly' approach, allowing you to adapt gradually and effectively to the changes you're implementing.

Remember, this is your pathway to better health. With persistence, self-advocacy and a commitment to holistic wellbeing, you can achieve meaningful and lasting improvements in managing migraine and enhancing your overall quality of life.

Future Improvements for You and Your Children

As you embark on your journey towards a healthier, pain-free future, let's revisit an important concept: epigenetics. We discussed earlier how epigenetics plays a pivotal role in migraine management. Lifestyle interventions such as dietary changes and regular exercise can influence how your genetic profile is expressed. These interventions have the potential to switch certain genes on or off, just like light switches in a room. In this way you are directly impacting the way your migraine presents.[2]

What's even more exciting, though, is that these positive changes don't stop with you. Through epigenetics, the improvements you make in your health can be passed on to your children, potentially reducing their likelihood of developing migraine or, at the very least, lessening their severity. By starting early, you're not only improving your own quality of life but also creating a healthier future for your children. Imagine someone like Chelsea, who comes from a long line of migraine sufferers, being able to break the cycle and positively influence her children's health through proactive lifestyle choices.

This is more than just changing your diet or exercising for your own benefit – it's about creating a legacy of health and wellbeing for the next generation. Epigenetics is set to become a cornerstone of future healthcare models, shifting the focus from merely managing symptoms to fostering long-term health and vitality.

Your Journey Begins Now

While the hope of transformation can be inspiring and motivating, I understand it may also feel frustrating if you're currently experiencing regular migraine episodes. It's important to acknowledge that your journey is unique, and the challenges you face are valid.

My goal in writing this book has been to help you better understand your migraine brain – why it reacts the way it does and how it leads to the painful symptoms that disrupt your daily life. More importantly, I hope this book has equipped you with the tools and knowledge to make meaningful changes that positively influence your brain pathways and overall health, enabling you to regain a sense of routine and control in your life.

You will find further guidance and resources, on my website www.mymigrainementor.com.au where I share my expertise as 'My Migraine Mentor'. This program is not theoretical – it is supported by research, which will no doubt continue to fine-tune and improve the process in the future.

As you embark on your own health journey, remember that every expedition begins with uncertainty. Your path may not have a clearly defined route or itinerary, but your destination is unmistakable: a life enriched with meaningful encounters, fulfilling social experiences and deep family connections. These are the moments that will bring greater satisfaction and purpose to your journey.

This is your time to write your own chapter – a story of resilience, growth and transformation. With each step forward, you are creating a narrative that reflects your strength and determination to live a life that is not defined by migraine but instead by the joy, connection and fulfilment you choose to embrace.

ONWARD

Reimagining Migraine Care

A Collaborative Holistic Approach

This book has been written with a clear focus on individuals who experience migraine – a condition that is not just a collection of symptoms but a disease with a genetic predisposition. The term 'disease' is fitting, as migraine creates a profound 'dis-ease' in the brain, which in turn affects the body. My hope is that this book has provided a balance of scientific insight to help you better understand your condition, alongside practical strategies to guide you towards improved health and wellbeing. Note more resources are available on www.mymigrainementor.com.au.

Beyond empowering individuals, I also hope this book sparks meaningful discussions and, more importantly, fosters collaboration among health professionals. Those who experience migraine – collectively, a group of people who require the support of a multidisciplinary team – deserve a healthcare approach that not only reduces migraine-related disability but also promotes long-term health benefits. The ultimate goal is to enable individuals to thrive, not just survive, and to live life to their fullest potential.

What Should Health Care for Migraine Look Like?

The United Nations' "2030 Agenda for Sustainable Development" provides a framework for promoting health equity worldwide. Recently, a group of headache specialists, primarily neurologists, explored how this agenda could be applied to headache treatment.[1] One of their key recommendations for migraine care is to adopt a biopsychosocial (BPS) perspective. This approach considers not only clinical features but also sociodemographic and lifestyle factors, such as socioeconomic status, work environment, habits, diet, sleep patterns, exercise and external stressors.

Currently, the western healthcare system remains heavily biased towards the medical model of treatment. In this model, patients often see a general physician or specialist who primarily focuses on prescribing medication as the first line of treatment. This approach is often driven by time constraints or the patient's desire for a quick fix. However, other pathways are available and should be explored.

When the BPS model was introduced by the World Health Organization (WHO) in 1948, allied health professions such as physiotherapy, psychology and dietetics were not as established as they are today. In 2025, we have a wealth of university-trained health professionals who are equipped with evidence-based knowledge to help rehabilitate individuals with various health conditions, including migraine. Despite their availability, these professionals remain underutilised in migraine care.

To shift from a reactive model – treating symptoms as they arise – to a proactive model that prioritises prevention, we need to adopt a team-based approach. Drawing from my experience in sports medicine, where multidisciplinary teams of physicians, surgeons, physiotherapists, dietitians, psychologists and exercise physiologists work together to optimise athletes' performance, I advocate for a similar model in migraine care. This collaborative approach can help individuals with migraine achieve their best possible health outcomes.

As I finalised this book, I came across an exciting publication called "Hallmarks of Primary Headache: Part 1 – Migraine".[2] This comprehensive review, authored by a diverse group of health professionals, including a physiotherapy colleague Matteo Castaldo, highlights the importance of broadening migraine treatment to include interventions such as diet, manual therapy, pain education and exercise. The authors emphasise the need for personalised care, tailored to each individual's unique circumstances – a perspective that aligns perfectly with the principles outlined in this book.

Castaldo, who is from Italy, shared that the collaborative process of creating this publication was challenging but ultimately rewarding, as it resulted in a more complete and comprehensive resource than any single professional could achieve alone. Similarly, a multidisciplinary approach to migraine care may present challenges, but the rewards for patients will undoubtedly be worth the effort.

Where Do We Begin?

The first step is to develop an intervention plan that incorporates lifestyle changes from the outset, rather than relying solely on medication. Consider the example of a heart patient who requires a stent, has high cholesterol, smokes and follows a poor diet. A cardiologist would likely recommend addressing lifestyle changes immediately, as well as starting medication following the surgical procedure. Lifestyle modifications would be encouraged and implemented as early as possible, and the same principle should apply to migraine care.

Research validates the urgency of addressing lifestyle factors in migraine management. Early intervention, driven by a cohesive medical team, can significantly improve outcomes. While funding and affordability may pose challenges, these can be mitigated by spreading costs over time.

Recognising migraine as a disease with significant global disability – particularly during the most productive years of life – should prompt health authorities to prioritise its management. Headaches, including migraine, are the leading cause of disability worldwide for individuals under 50, impacting not only the individual but also their families and communities.[3]

Solutions to this pressing issue may vary depending on geographic and systemic factors, but the need for change is universal. By embracing a collaborative, holistic and proactive approach to migraine care, we can empower individuals to lead healthier, more fulfilling lives.

The Future of Health Care

Achieving better health outcomes requires tailoring strategies to fit the unique healthcare systems of individual countries. For instance, Australia operates under a mixed public/private health model, while the United Kingdom leans heavily on a public system, and the United States is predominantly private. Each system has its own strengths and challenges. Regardless of the model, research consistently shows that investment in migraine care yields a positive cost-benefit analysis, even when using the traditional medical model. If we incorporate the biopsychosocial (BPS) model, which emphasises a more holistic approach, the returns could be even more significant.[4]

The transition from the traditional medical model to the BPS model is essential. While parts of the system have adopted elements of the BPS approach, it has yet to be implemented as a comprehensive, system-wide strategy. This shift requires setting broader health improvement goals alongside headache-specific goals, particularly when addressing comorbidities. It also demands a redistribution of responsibility, empowering individuals to take ownership of their health. This includes a combination of treatments such as medication, neck therapy, dietary adjustments, psychological support and aerobic fitness.

David Sinclair's book *Lifespan*[5] offers valuable insights into this approach. Sinclair, an Australian scientist, explores how diet, exercise and supplements can promote healthy ageing. His advocacy for shifting the focus from treating diseases to achieving health goals aligns perfectly with the principles of the BPS model. The interventions he emphasises – diet, exercise and supplementation – are consistent with the strategies needed to improve health outcomes for migraine sufferers.

Regardless of the healthcare model, effective communication among medical professionals is critical to developing a cohesive and efficient health strategy. Individual practitioners working in isolation cannot achieve the same level of success as a collaborative, multidisciplinary team. A unified approach ensures that all aspects of a patient's health are addressed, leading to better outcomes.

Overcoming Barriers

While the transition to a BPS model seems logical, it often feels like an insurmountable step. One major challenge is managing costs to ensure they remain sustainable for both individuals and governments. Proposals such as one-stop health centres have been suggested, but these may risk reducing patient autonomy. The ideal model will likely vary from country to country, reflecting the unique needs and resources of each healthcare system.

With many stakeholders involved in the process of change, finding the most effective model will be no easy path. It will also most likely vary significantly depending upon where you live. I had some insight into the process of change when reading the biography of Bono, the lead singer of U2.[6] He discussed his relentless efforts to transform the world's approach to a major health crisis – in his case it was AIDS. He had heard a story about Martin Luther King's approach to making change, even with people you don't always agree with. His goal was to find one aspect of a problem everyone could agree on; making change could then flow from that one point.

At the very least, as healthcare professionals involved in the treatment of migraine, we could all agree that striving for better health outcomes for every individual living with migraine is a truly commendable goal. This shared commitment would serve as the foundation for meaningful change within our current medical model for migraine care.

By starting with this common goal, we can begin to develop a healthcare system that not only provides relief for migraine sufferers but also enhances their overall health and resilience. As practitioners, we have an opportunity to be part of a healthcare model that prioritises holistic wellbeing over symptom management, supporting these individuals to lead productive, fulfilling lives.

Health professionals supporting individuals burdened by migraine can be well satisfied in knowing that their efforts have positively impacted someone's health journey. To me, contributing to improved wellbeing and quality of life is the most rewarding aspect – an indication of a job well done.

GLOSSARY

Acronymns Used In This Book

ACE – adverse childhood experience

ADD – attention deficit disorder

ADHD – attention deficit hyperactivity disorder

ANS – autonomic nervous system

BPS - biopsychosocial

CGH – cervicogenic headache

CCMI – Complete Concussion Management Inc.

CGRP – calcitonin gene-related peptide

CM – chronic migraine

CNS – central nervous system

CBF - cerebral blood flow

CD – celiac disease

CN – cranial nerve

CSD - cortical spreading depression

CVS – cyclic vomiting syndrome

DNA - deoxyribonucleic acid

EDS – Ehlers-Danlos syndrome

EEG - electroencephalogram

ENT – ear, nose & throat doctor

fMRI - functional Magnetic Resonance Imaging

HR - heart rate

HIIT - high intensity interval training

HPA Axis – hypothalamus-pituitary-adrenal axis

ICHD-3 - International Classification of Headache Disorders 3rd edition

IBS – irritable bowel syndrome

MHD – monthly headache days

MOH - medication overuse headache

MWA – migraine with aura

NRL – National Rugby League

QUT - Queensland University of Technology

SNS – sympathetic nervous system

PFC - prefrontal cortex

PNS – parasympathetic nervous system

PPCS – persistent post-concussion symptoms

PTH – post-traumatic headache

PTSD – post-traumatic stress disorder

TTH - tension type headache

TCN - trigemino-cervical nucleus

WHA - Watson Headache® Approach

WHO - World Health Organisation

Book References

References – Introduction

1. Tu S, Liew D, Ademi Z, Owen AJ, Zomer E. The Health and Productivity Burden of Migraines in Australia. *Headache.* 2020; 60(10):2291-2303.

2. Ashina M, Katsarava Z, Do TP, et al, Migraine: epidemiology and systems of care. *Lancet.* 2021; 397(10283):1485-1495.

3. Buse DC, Scher AI, Dodick DW, Reed ML, Fanning KM, Manack Adams A, Lipton RB. Impact of Migraine on the Family: Perspectives of People With Migraine and Their Spouse/Domestic Partner in the CaMEO Study. *Mayo Clin Proc.* 2016 Apr 25:S0025-6196(16)00126-9.

4. Tam ACT, Naik H, Trenaman L, Lynd L, Zhang W. Health-related quality of life among women and men living with migraine: a Canada-wide cross-sectional study. *J Headache Pain.* 2024 Oct 9;25(1):170.

References – Chapter 1

1. Human Genome Project – U.S. Department of Energy Genomic Science. Accessed 25th November 2023. https://genomicscience.energy.gov.

2. Amiri P, Kazeminasab S, Nejadghaderi SA, et al. Migraine: A Review on Its History, Global Epidemiology, Risk Factors, and Comorbidities. *Front Neurol.* 2022 Feb 23;12:800605.

3. Solomon S, Diamond S, Mathew N, Loder E. American headache through the decades: 1950 to 2008. *Headache.* 2008 May;48(5):671-7.

4. Seng EK, Parker A, Shapiro RE, Buse DC, Robbins MS and Lipton RB, Living in society, living with migraine: Editorial for the 2022 Members' Choice Award paper. *Headache.* 2023; 63:714-716

5. Headache Classification Committee of the International Headache Society (IHS) The International Classification of Headache Disorders, 3rd edition. *Cephalalgia.* 2018;38(1):1-211.

6. Sutherland HG, Albury CL, Griffiths LR. Advances in genetics of migraine. *J Headache Pain.* 2019;20(1):72.

7. Ziegler DK, Hur YM, Bouchard TJ Jr, Hassanein RS, Barter R. Migraine in twins raised together and apart. *Headache.* 1998;38(6):417-422.

8. Harder AVE, Terwindt GM, Nyholt DR, van den Maagdenberg AMJM. Migraine genetics: Status and road forward. *Cephalalgia.* 2023;43(2):3331024221145962.

9. Grangeon L, Lange KS, Waliszewska-Prosół M, et al. Genetics of migraine: where are we now? *J Headache Pain.* 2023;24(1):12. Published 2023 Feb 20.

10. Chalmer MA, Rasmussen AH; International Headache Genetics Consortium; Chronic migraine: Genetics or environment? *Eur J Neurol.* 2021;28(5):1726-1736.

11. Buse DC, Reed ML, Fanning KM, et al. Comorbid and co-occurring conditions in migraine and associated risk of increasing headache pain intensity and headache frequency: results of the migraine in America symptoms and treatment (MAST) study. *J Headache Pain.* 2020;21(1):23. Published 2020 Mar 2.

12. Jiang YJ, Fann CS, Fuh JL, et al. Genome-wide analysis identified novel susceptible genes of restless legs syndrome in migraineurs. *J Headache Pain.* 2022;23(1):39. Published 2022 Mar 29.

References – Chapter 2

1. Angeles Fernández-Gil M, Palacios-Bote R, Leo-Barahona M, Mora-Encinas JP. Anatomy of the brainstem: a gaze into the stem of life. *Semin Ultrasound CT MR.* 2010;31(3):196-219.

2. Skorobogatykh K, van Hoogstraten WS, Degan D, et al. Functional connectivity studies in migraine: what have we learned? *J Headache Pain.* 2019;20(1):108. Published 2019 Nov 20.

3. Charles A. The pathophysiology of migraine: implications for clinical management. *Lancet Neurol.* 2018;17(2):174-182.

4. Dodick DW. Migraine. *Lancet.* 2018;391(10127):1315-1330.

5. Hsiao FJ, Chen WT, Pan LH, et al. Dynamic brainstem and somatosensory cortical excitability during migraine cycles. *J Headache Pain.* 2022;23(1):21. Published 2022 Feb 5.

6. Schulte LH, May A. The migraine generator revisited: continuous scanning of the migraine cycle over 30 days and three spontaneous attacks. *Brain.* 2016;139(Pt 7):1987-1993.

7. Schulte LH, Mehnert J, May A. Longitudinal Neuroimaging over 30 Days: Temporal Characteristics of Migraine. *Ann Neurol.* 2020;87(4):646-651.

8. Schulte LH, Menz MM, Haaker J, May A. The migraineur's brain networks: Continuous resting state fMRI over 30 days. *Cephalalgia.* 2020;40(14):1614-1621.

9. Russo A, Coppola G, Pierelli F, et al. Pain Perception and Migraine. *Front Neurol.* 2018;9:576. Published 2018 Aug 2.

10. Messina R, Rocca MA, Colombo B, et al. Dysregulation of multisensory processing stands out from an early stage of migraine: a study in pediatric patients. *J Neurol.* 2020;267(3):760-769.

References – Chapter 3

1. Headache Classification Committee of the International Headache Society (IHS) The International Classification of Headache Disorders, 3rd edition. Cephalalgia. 2018;38(1):1-211.

2. Watson DH, Drummond PD. The Role of the Trigemino Cervical Complex in Chronic Whiplash Associated Headache: A Cross-Sectional Study. *Headache*. 2016;56(6):961-975.

3. Watson DH, Drummond PD. Head pain referral during examination of the neck in migraine and tension-type headache. *Headache*. 2012;52(8):1226-1235.

4. Satpute K, Bedekar N, Hall T. Headache symptom modification: the relevance of appropriate manual therapy assessment and management of a patient with features of migraine and cervicogenic headache – a case report. *J Man Manip Ther*. 2020;28(3):181-188.

5. Szperka C. Headache in Children and Adolescents. *Continuum (Minneap Minn)*. 2021;27(3):703-731.

6. Asuncion RMD, Al Khalili Y, Chopra P. Migraine Headache in Childhood. In: *StatPearls*. Treasure Island (FL): StatPearls Publishing; March 4, 2023.

7. Barnes N, Millman G, James E. Migraine headache in children. *Clin Evid*. 2006;(15):469-475.

8. Albers L, Kries RV, Straube A, et al. Age- and sex-specific first health care use for migraine in 2016 in children and adolescents from prospectively collected health insurance data in Germany. *Cephalalgia*. 2019;39(9):1156-1163.

9. Onofri A, Pensato U, Rosignoli C, et al. Primary headache epidemiology in children and adolescents: a systematic review and meta-analysis. *J Headache Pain*. 2023;24(1):8. Published 2023 Feb 14.

10. Gelfand AA. Infant Colic. *Semin Pediatr Neurol*. 2016;23(1):79-82.

11. Özge A, Faedda N, Abu-Arafeh I, et al. Experts› opinion about the primary headache diagnostic criteria of the ICHD-3rd edition beta in children and adolescents. *J Headache Pain*. 2017;18(1):109. Published 2017 Nov 23.

12. Pavkovic IM, Kothare SV. Migraine and Sleep in Children: A Bidirectional Relationship. *Pediatr Neurol*. 2020;109:20-27.

13. Nita SA, Teleanu RI, Bajenaru OA. The Role of Polysomnography in Identifying Sleep Disorders in Children with Migraine. *J Med Life.* 2020;13(1):64-67.

14. Anda R, Tietjen G, Schulman E, Felitti V, Croft J. Adverse childhood experiences and frequent headaches in adults. *Headache.* 2010;50(9):1473-1481.

15. Anto MM, Karvounides D, Magerman Lynch J, Chadehumbe M, Szperka CL. Implementing screening and treatment for adverse childhood experiences in pediatric patients with headache at the Children's Hospital of Philadelphia. *Headache.* 2023;63(7):965-967.

16. Sikorski C, Mavromanoli AC, Manji K, Behzad D, Kreatsoulas C. Adverse Childhood Experiences and Primary Headache Disorders: A Systematic Review, Meta-analysis, and Application of a Biological Theory. *Neurology.* 2023;101(21):e2151-e2161.

17. Anto M, Jaffee S, Tietjen G, Mendizabal A, Szperka C. Adverse Childhood Experiences and Frequent Headache by Adolescent Self-Report. *Pediatr Neurol.* 2021;121:51-55.

18. Hammond NG, Colman I, Orr SL. Adverse childhood experiences and onset of migraine in Canadian adolescents: A cohort study. *Headache.* 2022;62(3):319-328.

19. Mansuri F, Nash MC, Bakour C, Kip K. Adverse Childhood Experiences (ACEs) and Headaches Among Children: A Cross-Sectional Analysis. *Headache.* 2020;60(4):735-744.

20. Giza CC, Hovda DA. The new neurometabolic cascade of concussion. *Neurosurgery.* 2014;75 Suppl 4(0 4):S24-S33.

21. Ashina H, Porreca F, Anderson T, et al. Post-traumatic headache: epidemiology and pathophysiological insights. *Nat Rev Neurol.* 2019;15(10):607-617.

22. Lucas S, Hoffman JM, Bell KR, Walker W, Dikmen S. Characterization of headache after traumatic brain injury. *Cephalalgia.* 2012;32(8):600-606.

23. Complete Concussion Management Incorporated: – CCMI – https://completeconcussions.com Accessed on multiple occasions

24. Kothari SF, Eggertsen PP, Frederiksen OV, et al. Characterization of persistent post-traumatic headache and management strategies in adolescents and young adults following mild traumatic brain injury. *Sci Rep*. 2022;12(1):2209. Published 2022 Feb 9.

25. Patricios JS, Schneider KJ, Dvorak J, et al. Consensus statement on concussion in sport: the 6th International Conference on Concussion in Sport-Amsterdam, October 2022. *Br J Sports Med*. 2023;57(11):695-711.

26. World Health Organization (1992). International Classification of Diseases and Related Health Problems, 10th Revision. World Health Organization: Geneva.

27. Dodick DW. Migraine. Lancet. 2018;391(10127):1315-1330.

28. Li F, Lu L, Shang S, et al. Altered static and dynamic functional network connectivity in post-traumatic headache. *J Headache Pain*. 2021;22(1):137. Published 2021 Nov 13.

29. Aboghazleh R, Parker E, Yang LT, et al. Brainstem and Cortical Spreading Depolarization in a Closed Head Injury Rat Model. *Int J Mol Sci*. 2021;22(21):11642. Published 2021 Oct 28.

30. Dumkrieger G, Chong CD, Ross K, Berisha V, Schwedt TJ. Static and dynamic functional connectivity differences between migraine and persistent post-traumatic headache: A resting-state magnetic resonance imaging study. *Cephalalgia*. 2019;39(11):1366-1381.

31. Packard RC, Ham LP. Pathogenesis of posttraumatic headache and migraine: a common headache pathway? *Headache*. 1997;37(3):142-152.

32. El Baassiri MG, Raouf Z, Badin S, Escobosa A, Sodhi CP, Nasr IW. Dysregulated brain-gut axis in the setting of traumatic brain injury: review of mechanisms and anti-inflammatory pharmacotherapies. *J Neuroinflammation*. 2024;21(1):124. Published 2024 May 10.

33. Fu T, Liu L, Huang X, et al. Cerebral blood flow alterations in migraine patients with and without aura: An arterial spin labelling study. *J Headache Pain.* 2022;23(1):131. Published 2022 Oct 4. doi:10.1186/s10194-022-01501-0

34. Terry DP, Büttner F, Huebschmann NA, Gardner AJ, Cook NE, Iverson GL. Systematic Review of Pre-injury Migraines as a Vulnerability Factor for Worse Outcome Following Sport-Related Concussion. *Front Neurol.* 2022;13:915357. Published 2022 Jun 20.

35. Jo J, Berkner PD, Stephenson K, et al. Examining Acute Symptoms After Sport-Related Concussion in Collegiate Athletes With Preinjury Migraines. *Clin J Sport Med.* 2024;34(5):404-410.

36. Terry DP, Jo J, Williams KL, et al. Recovery After Sport-Related Concussion in Collegiate Athletes With Self-Reported Pre-Injury Migraines. *J Neurotrauma.* 2024;41(15-16):e1986-e1995.

37. Morgan CD, Zuckerman SL, Lee YM, et al. Predictors of Postconcussion syndrome after sports-related concussion in young athletes: a matched case-control study. *J Neurosurg Pediatr.* 2015;15(6):589-598.

38. Sufrinko A, McAllister-Deitrick J, Elbin RJ, Collins MW, Kontos AP. Family History of Migraine Associated With Posttraumatic Migraine Symptoms Following Sport-Related Concussion. *J Head Trauma Rehabil.* 2018;33(1):7-14.

References – Chapter 4

1. Thomas Jefferson Foundation – Monticello Website – https://www.monticello.org/research-education/thomas-jefferson-encyclopedia/knowledge-power-quotation/

2. Ziegler DK, Hur YM, Bouchard TJ Jr, Hassanein RS, Barter R. Migraine in twins raised together and apart. *Headache.* 1998;38(6):417-422.

3. Mulder EJ, Van Baal C, Gaist D, et al. Genetic and environmental influences on migraine: a twin study across six countries. *Twin Res.* 2003;6(5):422-431.

4. Nijs J, Wyns A, Hendrix J. The importance of stress in the paradigm shift from a tissue- and disease-based pain management approach towards multimodal lifestyle interventions for chronic pain. *Braz J Phys Ther.* 2024;28(2):101061.

5. Kimoto K, Aiba S, Takashima R, et al. Influence of barometric pressure in patients with migraine headache. *Intern Med.* 2011;50(18):1923-1928.

6. Martin GV, Houle T, Nicholson R, Peterlin A, Martin VT. Lightning and its association with the frequency of headache in migraineurs: an observational cohort study. *Cephalalgia.* 2013;33(6):375-383.

7. Kelman L, Rains JC. Headache and sleep: examination of sleep patterns and complaints in a large clinical sample of migraineurs. *Headache.* 2005;45(7):904-910.

8. Buse DC, Rains JC, Pavlovic JM, et al. Sleep Disorders Among People With Migraine: Results From the Chronic Migraine Epidemiology and Outcomes (CaMEO) Study. *Headache.* 2019;59(1):32-45.

9. Bertisch SM, Li W, Buettner C, et al. Nightly sleep duration, fragmentation, and quality and daily risk of migraine. *Neurology.* 2020;94(5):e489-e496.

10. Vgontzas A, Pavlović JM. Sleep Disorders and Migraine: Review of Literature and Potential Pathophysiology Mechanisms. *Headache.* 2018;58(7):1030-1039.

11. Li B, Cao Y, Yuan H, et al. The crucial role of locus coeruleus noradrenergic neurons in the interaction between acute sleep disturbance and headache. *J Headache Pain.* 2024;25(1):31. Published 2024 Mar 5.

12. Vittorini MG, Sahin A, Trojan A, et al. The glymphatic system in migraine and other headaches. *J Headache Pain.* 2024;25(1):34. Published 2024 Mar 11.

13. Erland LA, Saxena PK. Melatonin Natural Health Products and Supplements: Presence of Serotonin and Significant Variability of Melatonin Content. *J Clin Sleep Med.* 2017;13(2):275-281. Published 2017 Feb 15.

14. Okazaki Y, Yoshida S, Kashima S, Koike S, Matsumoto M. Impact of the 2018 Japan Floods on prescriptions for migraine: A longitudinal analysis using the National Database of Health Insurance Claims. *Headache.* 2022;62(6):657-667.

15. Buse DC, Gerstein MT, Houts CR, et al. Impact of the COVID-19 pandemic on people living with migraine: Results of the MiCOAS qualitative study. *Headache.* 2022;62(3):284-293.

16. Scieszka D, Jin Y, Noor S, et al. Biomass smoke inhalation promotes neuroinflammatory and metabolomic temporal changes in the hippocampus of female mice. *J Neuroinflammation.* 2023;20(1):192. Published 2023 Aug 22.

17. Gelfand AA. Infant Colic. *Semin Pediatr Neurol.* 2016;23(1):79-82.

18. Moavero R, Papetti L, Bernucci MC, et al. Cyclic vomiting syndrome and benign paroxysmal torticollis are associated with a high risk of developing primary headache: A longitudinal study. *Cephalalgia.* 2019;39(10):1236-1240.

19. Rothner AD. Migraine Variants in Children. *Pediatr Ann.* 2018;47(2):e50-e54.

20. Arzani M, Jahromi SR, Ghorbani Z, et al. Gut-brain Axis and migraine headache: a comprehensive review. *J Headache Pain.* 2020;21(1):15. Published 2020 Feb 13.

21. Aurora SK, Shrewsbury SB, Ray S, Hindiyeh N, Nguyen L. A link between gastrointestinal disorders and migraine: Insights into the gut-brain connection. *Headache.* 2021;61(4):576-589.

22. Sun S, Fan Z, Liu X, Wang L, Ge Z. Microglia TREM1-mediated neuroinflammation contributes to central sensitization via the NF-κB pathway in a chronic migraine model. *J Headache Pain.* 2024;25(1):3. Published 2024 Jan 5.

23. Strandwitz P. Neurotransmitter modulation by the gut microbiota. *Brain Res.* 2018;1693(Pt B):128-133.

24. Sudo N, Chida Y, Aiba Y, et al. Postnatal microbial colonization programs the hypothalamic-pituitary-adrenal system for stress response in mice. *J Physiol.* 2004;558(Pt 1):263-275.

25. Hindiyeh NA, Zhang N, Farrar M, Banerjee P, Lombard L, Aurora SK. The Role of Diet and Nutrition in Migraine Triggers and Treatment: A Systematic Literature Review. *Headache.* 2020;60(7):1300-1316.

26. Fila M, Chojnacki C, Chojnacki J, Blasiak J. Is an "Epigenetic Diet" for Migraines Justified? The Case of Folate and DNA Methylation. *Nutrients.* 2019;11(11):2763. Published 2019 Nov 14.

27. Beuthin J, Veronesi M, Grosberg B, Evans RW. Gluten-Free Diet and Migraine. *Headache.* 2020;60(10):2526-2529.

28. Torres-Ferrús M, Ursitti F, Alpuente A, et al. From transformation to chronification of migraine: pathophysiological and clinical aspects. *J Headache Pain.* 2020;21(1):42. Published 2020 Apr 29.

29. 29Pavelić AR, Zebenholzer K, Wöber C. Reconceptualizing autonomic function testing in migraine: a systematic review and meta-analysis. *J Headache Pain.* 2024;25(1):54. Published 2024 Apr 10.

30. Mehta D, de Boer I, Sutherland HG, et al. Alterations in DNA methylation associate with reduced migraine and headache days after medication withdrawal treatment in chronic migraine patients: a longitudinal study. *Clin Epigenetics.* 2023;15(1):190. Published 2023 Dec 12.

31. Cohen F, Bobker S. From diet to disasters, lifestyle factors can affect headaches and migraine. *Headache.* 2023;63(6):712-713.

32. La Touche R, Fierro-Marrero J, Sánchez-Ruíz I, et al. Prescription of therapeutic exercise in migraine, an evidence-based clinical practice guideline. *J Headache Pain.* 2023;24(1):68. Published 2023 Jun 7.

33. Irby MB, Bond DS, Lipton RB, Nicklas B, Houle TT, Penzien DB. Aerobic Exercise for Reducing Migraine Burden: Mechanisms, Markers, and Models of Change Processes. *Headache.* 2016;56(2):357-369.

34. Zhao R. Exercise mimetics: a novel strategy to combat neuroinflammation and Alzheimer's disease. *J Neuroinflammation*. 2024;21(1):40. Published 2024 Feb 2.

35. Bruijn N, van Lohuizen R, Boron M, et al. Influence of metabolic state and body composition on the action of pharmacological treatment of migraine. *J Headache Pain*. 2024;25(1):20. Published 2024 Feb 13.

36. Varkey E, Cider A, Carlsson J, Linde M. A study to evaluate the feasibility of an aerobic exercise program in patients with migraine. *Headache*. 2009;49(4):563-570.

37. Raffaelli B, Do TP, Chaudhry BA, Ashina M, Amin FM, Ashina H. Menstrual migraine is caused by estrogen withdrawal: revisiting the evidence. *J Headache Pain*. 2023;24(1):131. Published 2023 Sep 21.

38. Varlibas A, Erdemoglu AK. Altered trigeminal system excitability in menstrual migraine patients. *J Headache Pain*. 2009;10(4):277-282.

39. Maddahi A, Warfvinge K, Holm A, et al. Progesterone distribution in the trigeminal system and its role to modulate sensory neurotransmission: influence of sex. *J Headache Pain*. 2023;24(1):154. Published 2023 Nov 14.

40. Gosalia H, Moreno-Ajona D, Goadsby PJ. Medication-overuse headache: a narrative review. *J Headache Pain*. 2024;25(1):89. Published 2024 May 31.

41. Munksgaard SB, Bendtsen L, Jensen RH. Detoxification of medication-overuse headache by a multidisciplinary treatment programme is highly effective: a comparison of two consecutive treatment methods in an open-label design. *Cephalalgia*. 2012;32(11):834-844.

42. Martin PR. Triggers of Primary Headaches: Issues and Pathways Forward. *Headache*. 2020;60(10):2495-2507.

43. Donoghue S, Martin PR, Boucher G, et al, Migraineurs suspected triggers vs associations statistically determined using a digital platform, Cephalalgia. 2016 Vol. 36(1S) 1–185.

44. Peris F, Donoghue S, Torres F, Mian A, Wöber C. Towards improved migraine management: Determining potential trigger factors in individual patients. *Cephalalgia.* 2017;37(5):452-463.

45. Ashina M, Katsarava Z, Do TP, et al. Migraine: epidemiology and systems of care. *Lancet.* 2021;397(10283):1485-1495.

46. Buse DC, Scher AI, Dodick DW, et al. Impact of Migraine on the Family: Perspectives of People With Migraine and Their Spouse/Domestic Partner in the CaMEO Study. *Mayo Clin Proc.* Published online April 25, 2016.

47. Harder AVE, Terwindt GM, Nyholt DR, van den Maagdenberg AMJM. Migraine genetics: Status and road forward. *Cephalalgia.* 2023;43(2):3331024221145962.

References – Chapter 5

1. Matharu M, Katsarava Z, Buse DC, et al. Characterizing neck pain during headache among people with migraine: Multicountry results from the Chronic Migraine Epidemiology and Outcomes - International (CaMEO-I) cross-sectional study. *Headache.* 2024;64(7):750-763.

2. Peris F, Donoghue S, Torres F, Mian A, Wöber C. Towards improved migraine management: Determining potential trigger factors in individual patients. *Cephalalgia.* 2017;37(5):452-463.

3. Oguz Akarsu E, Baykan B, Ertas M, et al. The persistence versus interchangeability of migraine and tension-type headaches in a 5-year population-based validated survey. *Cephalalgia.* 2020;40(1):39-48.

4. Safiri S, Kolahi AA, Hoy D, et al. Global, regional, and national burden of neck pain in the general population, 1990-2017: systematic analysis of the Global Burden of Disease Study 2017. *BMJ.* 2020;368:m791. Published 2020 Mar 26.

5. Szperka C. Headache in Children and Adolescents. *Continuum (Minneap Minn).* 2021;27(3):703-731.

6. Özge A, Faedda N, Abu-Arafeh I, et al. Experts› opinion about the primary headache diagnostic criteria of the ICHD-3rd edition beta in children and adolescents. *J Headache Pain.* 2017;18(1):109. Published 2017 Nov 23.

7. Landgraf MN, von Kries R, Heinen F, Langhagen T, Straube A, Albers L. Self-reported neck and shoulder pain in adolescents is associated with episodic and chronic migraine. *Cephalalgia.* 2016;36(8):807-811.

8. Landgraf MN, Biebl JT, Langhagen T, et al. Children with migraine: Provocation of headache via pressure to myofascial trigger points in the trapezius muscle? - A prospective controlled observational study. *Eur J Pain.* 2018;22(2):385-392.

9. Torres-Ferrús M, Ursitti F, Alpuente A, et al. From transformation to chronification of migraine: pathophysiological and clinical aspects. *J Headache Pain.* 2020;21(1):42. Published 2020 Apr 29.

10. Calhoun AH, Ford S, Millen C, Finkel AG, Truong Y, Nie Y. The prevalence of neck pain in migraine. *Headache.* 2010;50(8):1273-1277.

11. Malick A, Strassman RM, Burstein R. Trigeminohypothalamic and reticulohypothalamic tract neurons in the upper cervical spinal cord and caudal medulla of the rat. *J Neurophysiol.* 2000;84(4):2078-2112.

12. Liang Z, Thomas L, Jull G, Minto J, Zareie H, Treleaven J. Neck pain associated with migraine does not necessarily reflect cervical musculoskeletal dysfunction. *Headache.* 2021;61(6):882-894.

13. Jull G, Amiri M, Bullock-Saxton J, Darnell R, Lander C. Cervical musculoskeletal impairment in frequent intermittent headache. Part 1: Subjects with single headaches. *Cephalalgia.* 2007;27(7):793-802.

14. Amiri M, Jull G, Bullock-Saxton J, Darnell R, Lander C. Cervical musculoskeletal impairment in frequent intermittent headache. Part 2: subjects with concurrent headache types. *Cephalalgia.* 2007;27(8):891-898.

15. Liang Z, Galea O, Thomas L, Jull G, Treleaven J. Cervical musculoskeletal impairments in migraine and tension type headache: A systematic review and meta-analysis. *Musculoskelet Sci Pract.* 2019;42:67-83.

16. Watson DH, Drummond PD. Head pain referral during examination of the neck in migraine and tension-type headache. *Headache.* 2012;52(8):1226-1235.

17. Marin JC, Gantenbein AR, Paemeleire K, Kaube H, Goadsby PJ. Nociception-specific blink reflex: pharmacology in healthy volunteers. *J Headache Pain.* 2015;16:87.

18. Thiele A, Klehr L, Strauß S, et al. Preventive treatment with CGRP monoclonal antibodies restores brain stem habituation deficits and excitability to painful stimuli in migraine: results from a prospective case-control study. *J Headache Pain.* 2021;22(1):149. Published 2021 Dec 11.

19. Ates MP, Ferik S, Pektezel LD, Guven H and Comoğlu SS. Changes in the blink reflex during migraine with aura and the inter-attack period. *Neurol Sci Neurophysiol* 2021; 38:105-10.

20. Casillo F, Sebastianelli G, Di Renzo A, et al. The monoclonal CGRP-receptor blocking antibody erenumab has different effects on brainstem and cortical sensory-evoked responses. *Cephalalgia.* 2022;42(11-12):1236-1245.

21. Watson DH, Drummond PD. Cervical referral of head pain in migraineurs: effects on the nociceptive blink reflex. *Headache.* 2014;54(6):1035-1045.

22. Jafari M, Bahrpeyma F, Togha M, Hall T, Vahabizad F, Jafari E. Can upper cervical manual therapy affect the blink reflex in subjects with migraine and neck pain? *J Man Manip Ther.* 2024;32(2):190-197.

23. Castien R, De Hertogh W. A Neuroscience Perspective of Physical Treatment of Headache and Neck Pain. *Front Neurol.* 2019;10:276. Published 2019 Mar 26.

24. Di Antonio S, Arendt-Nielsen L, Ponzano M, et al. Cervical musculoskeletal impairments in the 4 phases of the migraine cycle in episodic migraine patients. *Cephalalgia.* 2022;42(9):827-845.

25. Ferracini GN, Florencio LL, Dach F, et al. Musculoskeletal disorders of the upper cervical spine in women with episodic or chronic migraine. *Eur J Phys Rehabil Med.* 2017;53(3):342-350.

26. Schwarz A, Ziegeler C, Daneshkhah S, May A, Luedtke K. Predicting the outcome of the greater occipital nerve block - an observational study on migraine patients with and without musculoskeletal cervical impairment. *Cephalalgia.* 2021;41(1):78-89.

27. de Almeida Tolentino G, Lima Florencio L, Ferreira Pinheiro C, Dach F, Fernández-de-Las-Peñas C, Bevilaqua-Grossi D. Effects of combining manual therapy, neck muscle exercises, and therapeutic pain neuroscience education in patients with migraine: a study protocol for a randomized clinical trial. *BMC Neurol.* 2021;21(1):249. Published 2021 Jun 29.

28. Amons AL, Castien RF, van der Wouden JC, De Hertogh W, Dekker J, van der Horst HE. Manual therapy as a prophylactic treatment for migraine: design of a randomized controlled trial. *Trials.* 2019;20(1):785. Published 2019 Dec 27.

29. Raggi A, Leonardi M, Arruda M, et al. Hallmarks of primary headache: part 1 - migraine. *J Headache Pain.* 2024;25(1):189. Published 2024 Oct 31.

30. Moore CS, Sibbritt DW, Adams J. A critical review of manual therapy use for headache disorders: prevalence, profiles, motivations, communication and self-reported effectiveness. *BMC Neurol.* 2017;17(1):61. Published 2017 Mar 24.

31. Rist PM, Hernandez A, Bernstein C, et al. The Impact of Spinal Manipulation on Migraine Pain and Disability: A Systematic Review and Meta-Analysis. *Headache.* 2019;59(4):532-542.

32. Chaibi A, Tuchin PJ, Russell MB. Manual therapies for migraine: a systematic review. *J Headache Pain.* 2011;12(2):127-133.

33. Muñoz-Gómez E, Inglés M, Serra-Añó P, Espí-López GV. Effectiveness of a manual therapy protocol based on articulatory techniques in migraine patients. A randomized controlled trial. *Musculoskelet Sci Pract.* 2021;54:102386.

34. Bialosky JE, Bishop MD, Price DD, Robinson ME, George SZ. The mechanisms of manual therapy in the treatment of musculoskeletal pain: a comprehensive model. *Man Ther.* 2009;14(5):531-538.

35. Muñoz-Gómez E, Serra-Añó P, Mollà-Casanova S, et al. Potential Add-On Effects of Manual Therapy Techniques in Migraine Patients: A Randomised Controlled Trial. *J Clin Med.* 2022;11(16):4686. Published 2022 Aug 11.

36. Di Antonio S, Arendt-Nielsen L, Castaldo M. Cervical musculoskeletal impairments and pain sensitivity in migraine patients. *Musculoskelet Sci Pract.* 2023;66:102817.

37. Di Antonio S, Arendt-Nielsen L, Ponzano M, et al. Migraine patients with and without neck pain: Differences in clinical characteristics, sensitization, musculoskeletal impairments, and psychological burden. *Musculoskelet Sci Pract.* 2023;66:102800.

38. Szikszay TM, Hoenick S, von Korn K, et al. Which Examination Tests Detect Differences in Cervical Musculoskeletal Impairments in People With Migraine? A Systematic Review and Meta-Analysis. *Phys Ther.* 2019;99(5):549-569.

39. Di Antonio S, Arendt-Nielsen L, Ponzano M, et al. Cervical musculoskeletal impairments in the 4 phases of the migraine cycle in episodic migraine patients. *Cephalalgia.* 2022;42(9):827-845.

40. Tedeschi R, Pillastrini P, Pierangeli G, Favoni V, Cortelli P, Cevoli S. Is physiotherapy in migraines known to sufferers? A cross-sectional study. *Neurol Sci.* 2024;45(4):1669-1674.

41. Jafari M, Bahrpeyma F, Togha M, Vahabizad F, Hall T. The effects of upper cervical spine manual therapy on central sensitization and brainstem auditory evoked potentials in subjects with migraine and neck pain. *J Bodyw Mov Ther.* 2024;40:184-189.

42. Nijs J, Malfliet A, Roose E, et al. Personalized Multimodal Lifestyle Intervention as the Best-Evidenced Treatment for Chronic Pain: State-of-the-Art Clinical Perspective. *J Clin Med.* 2024;13(3):644. Published 2024 Jan 23.

References – Chapter 6

1. Henryk-Gutt R, Rees WL. Psychological aspects of migraine. *J Psychosom Res.* 1973;17(2):141-153.

2. Castro Zamparella T, Carpinella M, Peres M, et al. Specific cognitive and psychological alterations are more strongly linked to increased migraine disability than chronic migraine diagnosis. *J Headache Pain.* 2024;25(1):37. Published 2024 Mar 15.

3. Radecki D and Hull L, *Psychological Safety*, Red Hill Publishing, 2018

4. Nijs J, Malfliet A, Roose E, et al. Personalized Multimodal Lifestyle Intervention as the Best-Evidenced Treatment for Chronic Pain: State-of-the-Art Clinical Perspective. *J Clin Med.* 2024;13(3):644. Published 2024 Jan 23.

5. Dodick DW. Migraine. *Lancet.* 2018;391(10127):1315-1330.

6. Charles A. The pathophysiology of migraine: implications for clinical management. *Lancet Neurol.* 2018;17(2):174-182.

7. Hadjikhani N, Ward N, Boshyan J, et al. The missing link: enhanced functional connectivity between amygdala and visceroceptive cortex in migraine. *Cephalalgia.* 2013;33(15):1264-1268.

8. Burstein R, Potrebic S. Retrograde labeling of neurons in the spinal cord that project directly to the amygdala or the orbital cortex in the rat. *J Comp Neurol.* 1993;335(4):469-485.

9. Verhagen IE, van Casteren DS, de Vries Lentsch S, Terwindt GM. Effect of lockdown during COVID-19 on migraine: A longitudinal cohort study. *Cephalalgia.* 2021;41(7):865-870.

10. Zamir O, Yarns BC, Lagman-Bartolome AM, Jobanputra L, Lawler V, Lay C. Understanding the gaps in headache and migraine treatment with psychological and behavioral interventions: A narrative review. *Headache.* 2023;63(8):1031-1039.

11. Hubig LT, Smith T, Williams E, et al. Measuring interictal burden among people affected by migraine: a descriptive survey study. *J Headache Pain.* 2022;23(1):97. Published 2022 Aug 8.

12. Yao C, Zhang Y, Lu P, et al. Exploring the bidirectional relationship between pain and mental disorders: a comprehensive Mendelian randomization study. *J Headache Pain.* 2023;24(1):82. Published 2023 Jul 7.

13. Kruse JA, Seng EK. Changes in cognitive appraisal in a randomized controlled trial of mindfulness-based cognitive therapy for patients with migraine. *Headache.* 2023;63(10):1403-1411.

14. Falla K, Kuziek J, Mahnaz SR, Noel M, Ronksley PE, Orr SL. Anxiety and Depressive Symptoms and Disorders in Children and Adolescents With Migraine: A Systematic Review and Meta-analysis. *JAMA Pediatr.* 2022;176(12):1176-1187.

15. 15 Pistoia F, Salfi F, Saporito G, et al. Behavioral and psychological factors in individuals with migraine without psychiatric comorbidities. *J Headache Pain.* 2022;23(1):110. Published 2022 Aug 26.

16. McCracken HT, Lee AA, Smitherman TA. Headache and psychological variables as predictors of disability in individuals with primary headache disorders. *Headache.* 2023;63(9):1259-1270.

17. Lee HJ, Lee JH, Cho EY, Kim SM, Yoon S. Efficacy of psychological treatment for headache disorder: a systematic review and meta-analysis. *J Headache Pain.* 2019;20(1):17. Published 2019 Feb 14.

18. Dudeney J, Sharpe L, McDonald S, Menzies RE, McGuire B. Are psychological interventions efficacious for adults with migraine? A systematic review and meta-analysis. *Headache.* 2022;62(4):405-419.

19. Grazzi L, D'Amico D, Guastafierro E, et al. Efficacy of mindfulness added to treatment as usual in patients with chronic migraine and medication overuse headache: a phase-III single-blind randomized-controlled trial (the MIND-CM study). *J Headache Pain.* 2023;24(1):86. Published 2023 Jul 14.

References – Chapter 7

1. Rosignoli C, Ornello R, Onofri A, et al. Applying a biopsychosocial model to migraine: rationale and clinical implications. *J Headache Pain*. 2022;23(1):100. Published 2022 Aug 11.

2. Raffaelli B, Fitzek M, Overeem LH, Storch E, Terhart M, Reuter U. Clinical evaluation of super-responders vs. non-responders to CGRP(-receptor) monoclonal antibodies: a real-world experience. *J Headache Pain*. 2023;24(1):16. Published 2023 Feb 27.

3. Nijs J, Malfliet A, Roose E, et al. Personalized Multimodal Lifestyle Intervention as the Best-Evidenced Treatment for Chronic Pain: State-of-the-Art Clinical Perspective. *J Clin Med*. 2024;13(3):644. Published 2024 Jan 23.

4. Castro Zamparella T, Carpinella M, Peres M, et al. Specific cognitive and psychological alterations are more strongly linked to increased migraine disability than chronic migraine diagnosis. *J Headache Pain*. 2024;25(1):37. Published 2024 Mar 15.

5. Amiri P, Kazeminasab S, Nejadghaderi SA, et al. Migraine: A Review on Its History, Global Epidemiology, Risk Factors, and Comorbidities. *Front Neurol*. 2022;12:800605. Published 2022 Feb 23.

6. Solomon S, Diamond S, Mathew N, Loder E. American headache through the decades: 1950 to 2008. *Headache*. 2008;48(5):671-677.

References – Chapter 8

1. Domitrz I, Cegielska J. Magnesium as an Important Factor in the Pathogenesis and Treatment of Migraine-From Theory to Practice. *Nutrients*. 2022;14(5):1089. Published 2022 Mar 5.

2. Slavin M, Li H, Khatri M, Frankenfeld C. Dietary magnesium and migraine in adults: A cross-sectional analysis of the National Health and Nutrition Examination Survey 2001-2004. *Headache*. 2021;61(2):276-286.

3. Ramsden CE, Zamora D, Faurot KR, et al. Dietary alteration of n-3 and n-6 fatty acids for headache reduction in adults with migraine: randomized controlled trial. *BMJ*. 2021;374:n1448. Published 2021 Jun 30.

4. Faurot KR, Park J, Miller V, et al. Dietary fatty acids improve perceived sleep quality, stress, and health in migraine: a secondary analysis of a randomized controlled trial. *Front Pain Res (Lausanne)*. 2023;4:1231054. Published 2023 Oct 25.

5. Martami F, Togha M, Seifishahpar M, et al. The effects of a multispecies probiotic supplement on inflammatory markers and episodic and chronic migraine characteristics: A randomized double-blind controlled trial. *Cephalalgia*. 2019;39(7):841-853.

6. Pavelić AR, Zebenholzer K, Wöber C. Reconceptualizing autonomic function testing in migraine: a systematic review and meta-analysis. *J Headache Pain*. 2024;25(1):54. Published 2024 Apr 10.

7. Nijs J, Malfliet A, Roose E, et al. Personalized Multimodal Lifestyle Intervention as the Best-Evidenced Treatment for Chronic Pain: State-of-the-Art Clinical Perspective. *J Clin Med*. 2024;13(3):644. Published 2024 Jan 23.

8. Zamir O, Yarns BC, Lagman-Bartolome AM, Jobanputra L, Lawler V, Lay C. Understanding the gaps in headache and migraine treatment with psychological and behavioral interventions: A narrative review. *Headache*. 2023;63(8):1031-1039. doi:10.1111/head.14624

9. Radecki D and Hull L, *Psychological Safety*, Red Hill Publishing, 2018

10. Raggi A, Leonardi M, Arruda M, et al. Hallmarks of primary headache: part 1 - migraine. *J Headache Pain*. 2024;25(1):189. Published 2024 Oct 31.

11. L Erland & P Saxena, Melatonin Natural Health Products and Supplements: Presence of Serotonin and Significant Variability of Melatonin Content, Journal of Clinical Sleeps Medicine 2017, Feb 15:13(2): 275-281.

12. Irby MB, Bond DS, Lipton RB, Nicklas B, Houle TT, Penzien DB. Aerobic Exercise for Reducing Migraine Burden: Mechanisms, Markers, and Models of Change Processes. *Headache.* 2016;56(2):357-369.

13. Zhao R. Exercise mimetics: a novel strategy to combat neuroinflammation and Alzheimer's disease. *J Neuroinflammation.* 2024;21(1):40. Published 2024 Feb 2.

14. Bruijn N, van Lohuizen R, Boron M, et al. Influence of metabolic state and body composition on the action of pharmacological treatment of migraine. *J Headache Pain.* 2024;25(1):20. Published 2024 Feb 13.

15. Van Der Donckt J, Vandenbussche N, De Brouwer M, et al. Analysis of free-living daytime movement in patients with migraine with access to acute treatment. *J Headache Pain.* 2025;26(1):33. Published 2025 Feb 13.

16. Varkey E, Cider A, Carlsson J, Linde M. A study to evaluate the feasibility of an aerobic exercise program in patients with migraine. *Headache.* 2009;49(4):563-570.

17. Varkey E, Cider A, Carlsson J, Linde M. Exercise as migraine prophylaxis: a randomized study using relaxation and topiramate as controls. *Cephalalgia.* 2011;31(14):1428-1438.

18. Peris F, Donoghue S, Torres F, Mian A, Wöber C. Towards improved migraine management: Determining potential trigger factors in individual patients. *Cephalalgia.* 2017;37(5):452-463.

19. Gosalia H, Moreno-Ajona D, Goadsby PJ. Medication-overuse headache: a narrative review. *J Headache Pain.* 2024;25(1):89. Published 2024 May 31.

20. Mehta D, de Boer I, Sutherland HG, et al. Alterations in DNA methylation associate with reduced migraine and headache days after medication withdrawal treatment in chronic migraine patients: a longitudinal study. *Clin Epigenetics.* 2023;15(1):190. Published 2023 Dec 12.

21. Vuralli D, Ceren Akgor M, Gok Dagidir H, Gulbahar O, Yalinay M, Bolay H. Lipopolysaccharide, VE-cadherin, HMGB1, and HIF-1α levels are elevated in the systemic circulation in chronic migraine patients with medication

overuse headache: evidence of leaky gut and inflammation. *J Headache Pain.* 2024;25(1):23. Published 2024 Feb 19.

22. Munksgaard SB, Bendtsen L, Jensen RH. Detoxification of medication-overuse headache by a multidisciplinary treatment programme is highly effective: a comparison of two consecutive treatment methods in an open-label design. *Cephalalgia.* 2012;32(11):834-844.

23. Diener HC, Antonaci F, Braschinsky M, et al. European Academy of Neurology guideline on the management of medication-overuse headache. *Eur J Neurol.* 2020;27(7):1102-1116.

24. Grazzi L, D'Amico D, Guastafierro E, et al. Efficacy of mindfulness added to treatment as usual in patients with chronic migraine and medication overuse headache: a phase-III single-blind randomized-controlled trial (the MIND-CM study). *J Headache Pain.* 2023;24(1):86. Published 2023 Jul 14.

25. Raffaelli B, Do TP, Chaudhry BA, Ashina M, Amin FM, Ashina H. Menstrual migraine is caused by estrogen withdrawal: revisiting the evidence. *J Headache Pain.* 2023;24(1):131. Published 2023 Sep 21.

26. Witteveen H, van den Berg P, Vermeulen G. Treatment of menstrual migraine; multidisciplinary or mono-disciplinary approach. *J Headache Pain.* 2017;18(1):45.

27. Horwitz S, Stewart A. An Exploratory Study to Determine the Relationship between Cervical Dysfunction and Perimenstrual Migraines. *Physiother Can.* 2015;67(1):30-38.

References – Chapter 9

1. Rosignoli C, Ornello R, Onofri A, et al. Applying a biopsychosocial model to migraine: rationale and clinical implications. *J Headache Pain.* 2022;23(1):100. Published 2022 Aug 11.

2. Gallardo VJ, Gómez-Galván JB, Asskour L, et al. A study of differential microRNA expression profile in migraine: the microMIG exploratory study. *J Headache Pain.* 2023;24(1):11. Published 2023 Feb 17.

References – Author's Note

1. Martelletti P, Leonardi M, Ashina M, et al. Rethinking headache as a global public health case model for reaching the SDG 3 HEALTH by 2030. *J Headache Pain*. 2023;24(1):140. Published 2023 Oct 27.

2. Raggi A, Leonardi M, Arruda M, et al. Hallmarks of primary headache: part 1 - migraine. *J Headache Pain*. 2024;25(1):189. Published 2024 Oct 31.

3. Kothari SF, Jensen RH, Steiner TJ. The relationship between headache-attributed disability and lost productivity: 1. A review of the literature. *J Headache Pain*. 2021;22(1):73. Published 2021 Jul 17.

4. Tu S, Liew D, Ademi Z, Owen AJ, Zomer E. The Health and Productivity Burden of Migraines in Australia. *Headache*. 2020;60(10):2291-2303.

5. Sinclair DA & LaPlante MD, *Lifespan*, HarperCollins Publishing 2019

6. Bono, *Surrender*, Hutchinson Heinmann 2022

Recommended Reading List

1. Two eBooks that will expand your knowledge migraine and concussion:

***Migraine in Children* eBook**

www.mymigrainementor.com.au

***Concussion – Dispelling the Myths* eBook**

www.sydneyconcussioncentre.com.au

2. *Plum* by Brendan Cowell

This fictional book thoughtfully explores life after brain injury from multiple concussions, providing insights that foster deeper understanding and empathy.

3. *Psychological Safety* by Dan Radecki & Leonie Hull

Referenced in Chapter 6, this book offers valuable insights into creating a workplace that is both productive and safe for employees at all levels of an organisation.

4. *Migraine and Yellow Flags* by Trina Morris

Trina Morris from Brisbane, Queensland, is a WHA colleague who has written this short story about the psychological challenges of dealing with migraine. Two other short stories explore the challenges of photophobia (light sensitivity) in migraine and recovery from concussion. These are titled *Photophobia and Migraine* and *Offside: But Why the Red Card?*

5. *Surrender: 40 Songs, One Story* by Bono

In his autobiography, Bono details, among other things, his ongoing involvement in efforts to reduce the global impact of AIDS, particularly addressing the challenges posed by the significant stigma attached to the disease. Similarly, the battle to reduce the impact of migraine as a disease shares parallels, given the different but equally limiting stigma surrounding its causes and presentation.

6. *Lifespan – Why We Age and Why We Don't Have To* by Dr David Sinclair
Outlive – The Science & Art of Longevity by Dr Peter Attia

These two books explore the science and practical strategies for living to an older age while remaining healthy. David Sinclair's book focuses on the science and potential future directions of medicine as we deepen our understanding of the ageing process and its impact on health. In contrast, Peter Attia's book places greater emphasis on the practical steps we can take to maintain and improve our health as we age.

7. Social Media Feeds

Here are some social media feeds I find useful. Always remember to do your own research and consult your trusted migraine professionals regarding anything you learn on social media.

- **My Migraine Mentor** @mymigrainementor

  The social media site, aligned with this book, explores relevant research and gives practical tips on navigating life with migraine.

- **Sydney Headache and Migraine Centre** @headacheandmigrainecentre

Sydney Concussion Centre @sydneyconcussioncentre

Associated with our Sydney-based centres which offer face-to-face consultations, these online profiles are dedicated to keeping you informed about all facets of headache and concussion care.

- **The Migraine Dietitian** @the.migraine.dietitian

  Kelli Yates, a qualified dietitian, runs this feed, offering up-to-date scientific research and practical ideas for developing a diet that can positively impact your migraine presentation.

- **The Holistic Psychologist** @the.holistic.psychologist

  Dr Nicole LePera runs an excellent feed that explains complex psychological principles in an easy-to-digest format. While not specifically aimed at migraine, the concepts are universal and applicable to various psychological situations.

- **Dr Mark Hyman** @drmarkhyman

  Mark Hyman, a functional medicine doctor, manages a fantastic social media feed that encourages us to view health through a holistic lens. He challenges us to approach health as a lifestyle choice for the present, rather than relying solely on medical intervention in the future.

8. For Health Professionals

Angeles Fernández-Gil M, Palacios-Bote R, Leo-Barahona M, Mora-Encinas JP. Anatomy of the brainstem: a gaze into the stem of life. *Semin Ultrasound CT MR*. 2010;31(3):196-219.

While not an easy read, this article on brainstem anatomy and function offers excellent insights into how our nonconscious brain operates. It's the kind of article that keeps on giving – you could revisit it every few months for an entire year and still discover something new each time.

9. CHAMP – HEADACHE & MIGRAINE DISEASE LANGUAGE & IMAGE GUIDE 2018/19, Coalition for Headache And Migraine Patients. Version 1.1 (June 2019).

A guide to the ideal terminology for migraine disease, aimed at fostering understanding and compassion for those living with it. (Available for download online.)

Acknowledgements

This book has truly been a collaborative effort, and I want to take a moment to acknowledge everyone who has contributed to its creation.

First and foremost, to Janine, my partner in life for the past 40 years and in business for the past 33 years – this book is as much yours as it is mine. You endured the dark days of migraine with unwavering love and patience, offering me the support I needed. Your insights, drawn from years of conversations with headache and migraine patients, made the language of this book more accessible and relatable. Your contributions elevated it to a level I could not have achieved alone.

To Kelsey Garlick, the editor of this book – when it became clear that I desperately needed an editor to bring this project to life, we realised you had been there all along. As someone who experiences migraine and a patient of our business partner Andris, you understood both the debilitating nature of migraine and the hope that comes with effective interventions. Your systematic approach brought clarity, direction, and focus to a process that initially felt overwhelming. You were the perfect editor for this book at exactly the right time.

To my children and extended family, who have witnessed me at my worst, thank you for your unwavering support of our family business from the very beginning. Your encouragement and interest in this project have meant the world to me.

To my colleagues at Sydney Headache and Migraine Centre – after over 40 years as a physiotherapist, I deeply value the importance of working with a skilled and like-minded team. Our discussions and collaborative efforts to tailor ideas for our diverse clients have been instrumental in shaping many of the concepts in this book. A special thank you to our support staff, who are on the front lines, providing patients with the guidance and care they need as they navigate life with migraine. A heartfelt thanks to Lani Croaker, our resident social media guru, for designing the diagrams that bring this book to life.

To Dean Watson, the developer of the Watson Headache® Approach, and Jane Watson, the administrative powerhouse behind it – thank you for your mentorship, friendship, and the incredible impact you've had on my health and our headache practice. Your support has been invaluable to Janine and me.

To the extended Watson Headache® family – Roger O'Toole, Helen Tufui, Trina Morris, Julie Walters, Damien Cummins, Matteo Castaldo, and many others – it has been a privilege to learn and grow alongside you. Here's to continued research and progress in the field of migraine care.

To Leonie Hull and Dan Radecki, thank you for your contributions to Chapter 6. Your insights were enlightening, and I am confident readers will find them as valuable as I did.

To everyone who has been part of the journey to expand migraine treatment into a holistic, multidisciplinary approach, thank you. To A/Professor Raymond Schwartz, A/Professor William Huynh, A/Professor Dennis Cordato, and the team at Southern Neurology, I am grateful for the opportunity to collaborate on the holistic care of migraine clients. To Thomas Paavola, a dietitian with a special interest in migraine and concussion, thank you for helping so many of our clients improve their diet and overall health.

To the medical researchers, such as Dr Rob Smith and the team at QUT, who have dedicated decades to advancing our understanding of migraine

– your work has made a profound difference to countless lives. At a time when science is often undervalued, it is important to acknowledge the countless hours you've spent striving to improve the lives of those with migraine. The many references in this book represent a tiny fraction of the work that has been done and will undoubtedly pave the way for future advancements to transform the lives of those living with migraine.

To the friends and patients who have shown interest in this book's progress over the years – your encouragement has been a powerful motivator. Special thanks to Keri Aggett, Brent Rae, Ingrid Rieger, Merryn Moffat and Craig Wilson for reading drafts and offering valuable suggestions that helped shape the final version.

Thank you to all my friends who permitted their stories to be shared. Balancing scientific insights with personal narratives adds depth and context to a topic that might otherwise feel overly clinical.

To the thousands of patients we've worked with at Sydney Headache and Migraine Centre over the past 17 years – thank you for being part of the journey, trusting us with your care – and for being open to trying new and innovative approaches to improve your quality of life. Your courage and resilience have been a constant source of inspiration.

Finally, to my Mum and Dad, who have been my lifelong role models. My Dad, as a dentist, offered invaluable insights into working with individuals enduring pain and discomfort. Together, they led lives defined by empathy and service, imparting to our family – and countless others – the profound importance of helping those in need. They were role models in the Salvation Army church they were involved in for over seventy years. Mum's passing in 2018 was a profound loss, but Dad, now 98, continues to inspire with his humour and wisdom.

Your legacy will live on for generations to come.

About the Author

Physiotherapist Rob Wallis has dedicated the past 17 years to the holistic treatment of headache and migraine, both personally and professionally. A passionate advocate for exploring better ways to manage migraine beyond medication, Rob has combined his personal experiences with professional expertise to develop a comprehensive approach to care.

In 2008, Rob began treating clients with headaches in his physiotherapy practice. By 2011, he took his commitment a step further, founding Sydney Headache and Migraine Centre – the first physiotherapy practice in Sydney solely dedicated to headache treatment. Since then, his professional focus has been on helping individuals overcome the challenges of headache and migraine disability through a holistic and evidence-based approach.

Having experienced migraine and headaches throughout his life, Rob brings a deep sense of empathy to his work. He understands firsthand the daily struggles of living with migraine and combines this personal insight with a thorough understanding of the science behind the condition. His approach empowers individuals to take control of their health and embark on a transformative journey toward lasting change.

Living in the beachside suburb of Cronulla in Sydney's south, Rob embraces the importance of a healthy lifestyle and its profound impact on managing migraine. His dedication to holistic care and his belief in the power of lifestyle changes inspire his work as My Migraine Mentor, helping countless individuals reclaim their lives from the limitations of migraine.

www.ingramcontent.com/pod-product-compliance
Lightning Source LLC
LaVergne TN
LVHW100300210926
848480LV00003B/974
9781764545501